O$_2$xygen:

Nature's Most Important Dietary Supplement

by Stephen R. Krauss

O₂xygen: Nature's Most Important Dietary Supplement

Copyright © 1999
BIO2 Publishing Company
First Printing 1999

ISBN: 0-7392-1115-8
Library of Congress Catalog Card Number: 99-94058

Published by:
BIO2 International, Inc.
San Luis Obispo, CA 93405
(805) 549-0275 / fax - (805) 549-9790
e-mail: bio2@ix.netcom.com

Printed in the U.S.A. by
Morris Publishing
3212 E. Highway 30 - Kearney, NE 68847

Acknowledgments:

This book is dedicated to my wife, Sherrie Lynn, for her continued faith, patience and counsel. Without her encouragement I never would have devoted the time and energy into this project as well as investing my talents in the field of oxygen supplementation. I would also like to thank Calvin Smith for sharing his wisdom and the numerous hours of stories that formed the real historical background for my search to find the truth about oxygen supplements. Lastly, I would humbly like to thank the countless numbers of individuals who let me into their personal lives concerning their health challenges and how they benefitted from oxygen therapies. They are the true pioneers and the ones who have suffered greatly, never faltering in their hope to find relief from their infirmities.

Author's Note:

The data and references provided and quoted in this book are based on research, experiments and information believed to be accurately and reliably reported for the applications described. However, no warranty is made, neither expressed nor implied, regarding the accuracy of the obtained results from the use of such data. The author will assume no responsibility for the results nor the performance of products and applications over which the author has no control. The author has made every effort to keep the information as generic as possible by eliminating all references to trade-named products and has replaced all such names with the phrase "stabilized oxygen". Numbers in parenthesis "(26)" which occur throughout the book refer to authors and articles which are listed in Appendix IX (Annotated Bibliography).

Table of Contents

Foreword:

Dr. Eldon Wayne Askew, Ph.D.
Professor and Director
Division of Foods and Nutrition
University of Utah

Oxygen? A dietary supplement? Can one "breathe" dietary supplements? Prior to reading Stephen R. Krauss' book, *Oxygen: Nature's Most Important Dietary Supplement,* I had not given much consideration to the concept of oxygen as a "nutrient". An essential element for the support of life, certainly, but hardly in the category of "classical" food-borne nutrients such as vitamin C, iron, calcium and protein.

Steve is, however, not proposing to supplement one's oxygen supply by inhaling bottled oxygen. He suggests you drink it, dissolved in water. Oxygen consumed in this way does seem to approach our traditional definition of an essential nutrient: a chemical organic or inorganic substance present in food and necessary for life which cannot be synthesized in the body in adequate amounts for optimum health or body functions. I was interested and read further.

My own interests in fuel metabolism at high altitudes and what Steve seemed to be saying about oxygen lead me to ask: "What would be the effect on

7

human performance in oxygen-poor environments if significant amounts of stabilized dissolved oxygen were ingested in water?" By the conservative and classical nature of academic training, most scientists are rather skeptical of dietary supplements promising unbelievable results.

Steve has, however, managed to assemble enough information on the issue of oxygen therapy to be at the least thought-provoking to most skeptics, including myself. After a number of phone calls with Steve, and after meeting with him at the University with my colleagues to discuss the potential uses of stabilized oxygen and possible research projects, I was intrigued by the concept of providing dissolved oxygen via the digestive tract as a potential means to circumvent the limitations of overtaxed hemoglobin molecules and oxygen-starved tissues especially during exhaustive exercise at higher altitudes.

There is no question that oxygen is absolutely essential to life. Professor J.S. Haldane devoted his life to the study of the behavior of gasses such as oxygen. In 1920, he communicated the following to his colleague Sir Joseph Barcroft: "Anoxemia (a critical lack of oxygen) not only stops the (human) machine, but wrecks the machinery (organ systems)." The comments in parenthesis are mine.

I borrowed this quote from an article by Dr. W.L. Krause, M.D., "Does exposure to altitude impair neurological function?" which appeared in Wilderness Medicine Newsletter [11(3) 1, 1994] because it illustrates the pervasive importance of oxygen. Oxygen transport and utilization are the result of several physiological processes including ventilation, hemoglobin affinity, cardiac output, blood flow, oxygen diffusion and extraction by the tissue (such as muscle), and ultimately its participation in oxidative metabolism.

Metabolism is much more efficient in the presence of adequate amounts of oxygen. Hence, physiological restrictions abound when oxygen becomes limiting. Increased extraction of oxygen from the blood by tissues during adaptation to hypoxia, (a lack of sufficient body oxygen for normal metabolic functions,) is one of the major adaptive mechanisms of the human body faced with the difficult task of coping with the breathing of "thin" air.

High altitude natives such as the Himalayan Sherpas and the Andean Quechuas have adapted to lifetimes of living in "thin" air. They have become very efficient utilizers of oxygen at reduced atmospheric pressures. Those of us who are confined to less lofty climates sometimes attempt to cram a lifetimes of Sherpa and Quechua adaptations into a week of vacation skiing at moderate altitudes.

The price we lowland natives pay for our indulgence is usually two to three days of headaches, nausea and malaise before some acute adaptations to altitude begin to "kick in" and help us cope with this environment of reduced oxygen tension. Even if we don't experience the effects of acute altitude illness, our oxygen-starved lungs and muscles are likely to notice a significant difference in the level of exertion at altitude whether we are skiing, climbing, backpacking or just hiking in the mountains.

Imagine, (and this is pure conjecture on my part,) that you could carry a convenient oxygen supply along with you that could serve the dual purpose of providing both hydration and supplemental oxygen. Would drinking copiously from a bottle of oxygen-enriched water help those hypoxia-impaired hemoglobin molecules by boosting the amount of dissolved oxygen in the blood and tissues? At the very least, this elixir should help prevent dehydration from altitude-induced diuresis and would be a lot more convenient than carrying around a bottle of oxygen gas and a mask!

Many questions remain to be answered concerning the potential benefits of oxygen enriched water. However, this does not dampen my enthusiasm for the potential applications of oxygen as a "dietary supplement". Would oxygen enriched water actually benefit physical or mental performance at sea level or altitude? Do unforeseen hazards exist regarding chronic use of oxygen enriched products?

Frankly, I do not know, but I would like to find out. This seems to be a very fertile area for additional scientific research. A supplement that would help prevent the "wrecking" of our internal body chemistry under conditions of oxygen deficit would be beneficial, indeed.

Is stabilized oxygen, Vitamin "O" as it has been described as, beneficial in that regard? I remain a cautiously enthused skeptic. You can make up your own mind after you read *Oxygen: Nature's Most Important Dietary Supplement.*

E. Wayne Askew, Ph.D.

Dr. Askew is currently a professor and the Director of the Division of Foods and Nutrition at the University of Utah. He has a Ph.D. in nutritional biochemistry, an M.S. in nutrition and a B.S. in agricultural science. Prior to his tenure at the University of Utah, Dr. Askew was the Chief, Military Nutrition Division for the U.S. Army Research Institute of Environmental Medicine and the Department of Defense's (D.O.D.) representative to the U.S. Interagency Committee on Human Nutrition Research and Interagency Board on Nutrition Monitoring and Related Research. He has also served as the Chief of the U.S. Army's Biochemistry Service, Radioisotope Services, and Chief, Lipid Research Branch, Chemistry Division. His specialty is Environmental Medicine, Exercise, Nutrition and Oxidative Stress.

Introduction:

Almost five years ago, I received a bottle of a solution that the manufacturer claimed would bring tremendous healing benefits to the body. The product literature stated that the liquid being sold contained high concentrations of stabilized oxygen which would not only destroy infectious microbes but would improve metabolism.

I was both interested and skeptical. I wanted to learn more. Certainly oxygen is the key factor in sustaining life. But ingesting oxygen and somehow that same oxygen getting into the blood stream was another story. Having spent as many years as I have in marketing and sales, one thing I know is that product claims must be substantiated by credible sources.

Getting my hands on detailed scientific information that described the processes, chemical contents and the efficacy of this and other oxygen-rich supplements was nearly impossible. And so began my quest for the truth about stabilized oxygen which eventually led me to general research about oxygen and its function and importance to living organisms.

Oxygen was independently discovered by the Swedish pharmacist (apothecary) Karl Scheele in 1772 and the English amateur chemist Joseph Priestly in 1775. Priestly called oxygen "dephlogisticated air" and after isolating it and breathing it he felt that it was "peculiarly beneficial." He wrote, some 222 years ago: "Who can tell, but that, in time, this pure air may become a fashionable article in luxury. Hitherto, only two mice and myself have had the privilege of breathing it." (52)

From Priestly to today, thousands of articles have been written in medical journals throughout the world defining oxygen's importance in maintaining and sustaining life. No other element has been surrounded with as much controversy. Life cannot exist without it and yet, because of its capacity to oxidize -- or share electrons -- with virtually every other element that exists, oxygen does have a "darker side".

This book is not intended to be a science book, medical journal or compendium on oxygen and its medicinal use since oxygen was discovered back in 1772. Instead, this book started out as simply a file of articles, studies and testimonials for my own personal use. But because the information was so diverse and, as I soon discovered, the facts surrounding oxygen therapies so misunderstood and misquoted, I soon discovered a growing need to put these materials in a book that anyone could read and understand.

The more I have learned about oxygen, its beneficial healing properties, its ability to cleanse, disinfect and improve health, the more I am convinced that it is not here on the earth by pure chance. There is a divinely inspired interaction between oxygen-producing plant life and oxygen-consuming higher life forms. A reduction in oxygen levels on our planet of even a few percentage points can adversely affect this delicate balance which maintains life or causes it to die out. Only mankind, of all the thousands of species that exist, has the ability to drastically alter this balance.

Certainly history has already shown that, because of our global irresponsibility, ignorance and complacency, we have already damaged the quality of the oxygen supply on this planet that we have been entrusted to protect. Our mutual responsibility is great if we are to leave a legacy of clean air with healthy oxygen levels to our children and their children.

Stephen R. Krauss
San Luis Obispo, California

Disclaimer:

This book is a compilation and summary of research that was conducted over a twenty-five year period on a variety of stabilized oxygen supplements by professionals in numerous disciplines as well as independent professional testing laboratories, colleges and universities throughout the world.

The following information has been obtained by or was provided to the author both in written as well as verbal format by individuals, testing facilities and consumers concerning their independent observations as to the benefits of stabilized oxygen products.

This information is not intended to recommend oxygen supplements as drugs, as a diagnosis for specific illnesses or conditions, nor as products to eliminate diseases or other medical conditions or complications. Rather, it is intended to provide an historical background on the combined data currently available on stabilized oxygen supplements.

The author makes no medical claims as to the benefits of stabilized oxygen to improve the medical condition of individuals.

The author recommends that individuals discuss all medical interests, diagnostic, or physiological concerns with a qualified physician or practitioner prior to purchasing and taking any oxygen-based supplement.

Please also note that most stabilized oxygen supplements are normally sold as vitamin (dietary) supplements in the United States under the F.D.A.'s Dietary and Supplement Health Education Act (D.S.H.E.A.) and are not sold as prescription pharmaceuticals nor as over-the-counter drugs.

Chapter One:

An Introduction to Oxygen As A Nutritional Dietary Supplement

"Oxidation is the source of life. Its lack causes impaired health or disease; its cessation, death."

Dr. Eugene Blass, Ph.D.
"Oxygen Therapy: Its Foundation, Aim & Result"

For almost 225 years, researchers and health practitioners have observed that patients using all forms of oxygen-based therapies (including stabilized oxygen supplements) have experienced improved health and well-being. The first recorded application of oxygen in treating a patient occurred in 1783 and was administered by the French physician Caillens. (45) Since that time, oxygen -- as a therapeutic treatment -- has been well researched and its benefits documented by thousands of experts in various medical and scientific disciplines.

Perhaps the most detailed chronological and annotated overview on "supplemental oxygen" therapies was compiled by Dr. Lawrence Martin, M.D., Chief, Division of Pulmonary and Critical Care Medicine at Mt. Sinai Medical Center in Cleveland, Ohio U.S.A. In his published article "Oxygen Therapy: The First 150 Years", Dr. Martin wrote in his introduction:

"Although oxygen's life-supporting role was understood early on, it took about 150 years for the gas to be used in a proper fashion for patients. For the first 150 years after discovery, therapeutic use of oxygen was sporadic, erratic, controversial. comical, beset by quackery, and only occasionally helpful. Not until the pioneering work of Haldane, Stadie, Barcroft and others, early in the 20th century, was oxygen therapy placed on a rational, scientific basis." (45)

How can the most abundant element on the earth provide such remarkable physiological benefits? To answer this question, we first have to understand just what oxygen is and how important oxygen is to a healthy body.

Simple Oxygen Chemistry

Oxygen is one of the five basic elements of all life (oxygen, hydrogen, carbon, nitrogen and sulphur) and is colorless, tasteless and odorless. None of these five basic elements, or any other element for that matter, is as abundant as oxygen. In addition, only oxygen is capable of combining with almost every other element and is essential in combustion.

The earth's crust is estimated to be 49.2% oxygen by weight; oxygen constitutes almost 85% of sea water, 47% of dry soil, 42% of all vegetation, 46% of igneous rocks and over 65% of the human body.

The two men credited with the discovery of oxygen in 1773 are the Swedish pharmacist Karl Wilhelm Scheele and English chemist Joseph Priestly. But it wasn't until 1777 that the French chemist and scientist Antoine Laurent Lavoisier demonstrated that oxygen was a pure substance and a component of air.

The most common and stable form of oxygen is diatomic oxygen, or "O_2". This is the primary molecular oxygen form used by all living creatures taken in by respiration. Other forms of oxygen, like singlet oxygen "O_1" and ozone "O_3", are more reactive and quickly combine with, or "oxidize", other atoms or molecules to form new compounds. It is oxygen's "reactive" nature that makes it so remarkable and beneficial.

Oxygen-The Basis For All Life

No other element is as important as atomic oxygen (with its eight electrons per atom.) Oxygen is absolutely critical to the life processes of all living creatures. According to medical research, 80% of the aerobic metabolic energy we need in our bodies comes from aerobic metabolism linked to oxygen with only 10% of our energy coming from food without further metabolism. This energy production is directly related to the consumption of high energy phosphate compounds that occur in foods that contain adenosine tri-phosphate/A.T.P., (see Chapter Three for more information about A.T.P.,) and creatine phosphate.

Current scientific measurements of the air we breathe indicates that oxygen levels are about 20% by volume. The remainder is hydrogen, nitrogen (the greatest component of air) and other toxic and non-toxic gasses. Interestingly enough, some scientists now believe that the levels of atmospheric oxygen were substantially higher when the earth was younger, as high as 50% according to some researchers. This theory was further substantiated in an Associated Press release article discussing why the dinosaurs disappeared:

> "Dinosaurs weren't done in by a giant asteroid, as one theory holds, but by a change in the atmosphere that meant there wasn't enough oxygen to support their inefficient respiratory systems..." (20)

Additionally, measurements of the oxygen levels of our air indicate a decline since the advent of the Industrial Revolution. Some medical professionals believe that the decline in atmospheric oxygen may be one of the causes of increased illness and the spread of many infectious diseases. (We'll talk about oxygen's remarkable disinfecting "power" a bit later in the book!)

Oxygen is brought to the lungs by respiration where it diffuses from the air into the blood stream through more than 140 square meters of internal lung surface area called the "gastric mucosa". Each lung has over 300 million alveolar sacs which look like clusters or bunches of grapes. If these were flattened out and connected together they would make a surface area of about 260 square feet.

The average individual takes in approximately 6 liters of air per minute, (about 14 breaths per minute - - 800 quarts per hour -- some 15,000 times each day,) during what is called a "resting state". Under heavy exertion or stress, this rate can increase from six to more than 15 liters per minute.

Oxygen from the lungs rapidly diffuses into the blood plasma from the alveolar sacs into the capillaries that surround them because the membranes of the alveoli are so thin that the oxygen molecules can pass right through them. As these life-giving oxygen molecules diffuse into the blood stream, they bind to the hemoglobin molecules in the iron-rich red blood cells.

As the hemoglobin molecule accepts oxygen, it releases carbon dioxide which then follows the opposite path that oxygen takes into the blood stream and so is eventually released back out of the lungs as a waste gas. This exchange of gasses is what is called respiration.

The hemoglobin molecules on each red blood cell become over 95% saturated with the available oxygen where this oxygen is then carried and eventually transferred to every one of the billions of cells in our bodies. The oxygen, once in these "recipient" cells is consumed as sugars, fats and protein are converted to energy and heat. The more energy or warmth our body needs, the more oxygen that is consumed.

This process is called "oxidation" and carbohydrates (sugars), fats and proteins (substrates) are what are oxidized (or "burned") for the body's fuel. Therefore the cells, to remain healthy and to continue to perform their function of providing energy for the body, must have an adequate and continuous supply of oxygen. The lower the oxygen content of the body, the less the body is able to oxidize substrates and to detoxify itself.

Mineral deficiencies contribute to oxygen depletion, especially a lack of iron which is the only mineral whose sole function is to secure oxygen to each and every red blood cell. A lack of chromium affects blood sugar concentrations and sugar (glucose) is essential in energy production. Cobalt is important to red blood cell production. Copper is required as a catalyst to store and release iron. Magnesium and phosphorus are also involved in energy production. Manganese is a key component of the oxygen-handling enzymes.

Many foods form acids in the body and may temporarily reduce our oxygen and mineral reserves. These include flesh foods, refined grains, soft drinks, carbonated drinks and alcoholic beverages.

Do we get enough oxygen into our blood stream? And if we don't, what happens to our cells and vital organs when they are denied an adequate supply of oxygen? These are vital questions that scientists and researchers have debated for many years. At the heart of their search for answers is the intricate and important functioning of the blood stream, the "river of life" which is the transport system for nutritional oxygen.

Chapter Two:

The Blood Stream...
The River of Life

*"Oxygen is needed in the body.
We can be without food and water
for a lengthy time.
We can be without oxygen
only for a few seconds.
It is the spark of life."*

**Dr. Charles H. Farr, M.D., Ph.D.
O2 Therapies**

Human blood has three main components: plasma, white blood cells and red blood cells. Our blood will settle into three distinct layers if left in a test tube. The red blood cells, the most numerous in the blood stream, will settle on the bottom. White blood cells, including lymphocytes, monocytes, eosinophils, basophils, neutrophils, and platelets, will form a thin white line in the middle. A deep, yellowish, watery plasma will float to the top.

Plasma is the actual "river" in which all the working constituents of our blood are carried in our remarkable circulatory system. Among the many constituents in this river is dissolved oxygen - up to 5% can be dissolved in this fluid. Unlike fish that can exist only on this dissolved oxygen in the plasma stream, the human body requires more oxygen than the plasma can provide. This is why red blood cells

Anatomy of Blood:
The River of Life

The Plasma: A yellow-colored saline liquid consisting mainly of 95% water , 3% oxygen as well as dissolved nutrients, waste products, proteins and hormones. Nutrients include sugars, fats, amino acids, vitamins and minerals. The waste products are the end result of cellular metabolism and include Uric acid (from the breakdown of DNA and RNA in the cells,), carbon dioxide and bilirubin (from the breakdown of red blood cells). Proteins include enzymes, antibodies and hemoglobin. Hormones include a variety of chemicals that control bodily functions including growth and sexual development.

The Blood: Almost half the volume of blood consists of cells. These include red blood cells (erythrocytes), white blood cells (leukocytes) and platelets (thrombocytes). Red blood cells transport oxygen to the cells where it is exchanged with carbon dioxide. White blood cells protect the body against infection and include granulocytes, monocytes and lymphocytes. Platelets help stop bleeding.

are so important since their role is to carry tremendous amounts of oxygen to the tissues in our body. But these red blood cells also get some of their oxygen from the plasma.

The body, in its own remarkable way, does not allow all of the red blood cells' oxygen to be consumed as it courses through our bodies. Under normal conditions, 70% to 75% of the oxygen that starts the journey in the red cells completes the return trip to the lungs. Thus, from 5% to as much as 50% of the oxygen is consumed by normal cellular metabolism. If, however, the body undergoes exertion, stress, illness or any other prolonged physical activity, this "reserve" can drop to 20% to 25%. Dr. Arthur Guyton, M.D., and author of the most widely accepted text on Medical Physiology wrote:

"Normally, about 97% of the oxygen transported from the lungs to the tissues is carried in chemical combination with hemoglobin in the red blood cells, and the remaining three percent in the dissolved state in the water of the plasma and the cells...

"The fraction of the blood that gives up its oxygen as it passes through the tissue capillaries is called the *utilization coefficient*. Normally, this is approximately 0.25, or 25% of the blood...During strenuous exercise, as much as 75% to 85% of the blood can give up its oxygen...However, in local tissue areas where the blood flow is very slow or the metabolic rate very high, utilization coefficients approaching 100% have been recorded -- that is, essentially all the oxygen is removed." (25)

It seems obvious that, if you can raise the amount of oxygen dissolved in the plasma, primarily at the lung alveolar interface as well as at other sites, you will also increase the amount of oxygen that gets to the cells and that can become a part of the oxygen "reserve". (Keep this principle in mind as we discuss oxygen supplements later in the book.)

The red blood cells, as carriers or the transportation system for oxygen, gather oxygen from the plasma and deliver this much needed oxygen to the capillaries where it is released again into the plasma for the cells to use to create the energy they need for healthy cellular metabolism.

Chapter Three:

How Do Cells Get Their Energy?

"Cancer cells originate from normal body cells in two phases. The first phase is the irreversible injuring of respiration. Just as there are many remote causes of plague -- heat, insects, rats -- but only one common cause, the plague bacillus, there are a great many remote causes of cancer -- tar, rays, arsenic, pressure, urethane -- but there is only one common cause into which all other causes of cancer merge, the irreversible injuring of respiration."

Dr. Otto Warburg
The Origin of Cancer Cells,
Science (1956)

Dr. Otto Warburg is still recognized as one of the premier experts on cellular metabolism and how and why healthy cells need oxygen to create the "energy" for all life processes. (Dr. Warburg received a Nobel Peace Prize for Medicine based on his research findings on the importance of oxygen to cellular life in 1931 and a second Nobel Prize in 1944 for his discovery of the hydrogen transferring enzymes! He was, until his retirement, the Director of the Max Planck Institute for Cell Physiology in Berlin, Germany. The complete text of his lecture delivered before the German Central Committee for Cancer Control in Stutt-

The Metabolic Process:

How our cells create energy using oxygen.

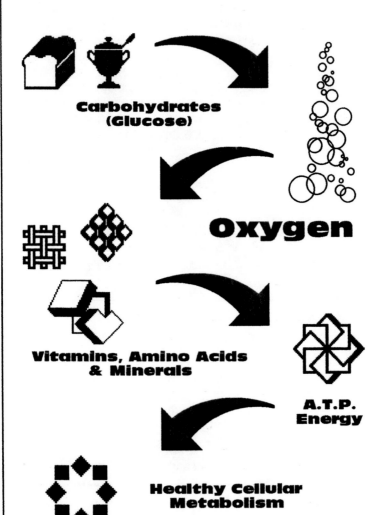

Carbohydrates
(Glucose)

Oxygen

Vitamins, Amino Acids
& Minerals

A.T.P.
Energy

Healthy Cellular
Metabolism

How the Body Creates Energy!

Glucose molecules (from complex carbohydrates) in the cell are made up of carbon, hydrogen and oxygen atoms. Glucose, along with other energy-yielding substrates, is the "FUEL" for the cells' energy production. Oxygen (O2) is necessary for the aerobic combustion of glucose in each cell.

As the glucose fuel is "burned" the cells create adenosine triphosphate (ATP) the source of power for all cell, organ and body functions. This is a naturally occurring process. During the burning of the glucose and the formation of ATP, free radicals are naturally created. The body is designed to diffuse and eliminate these free radicals with anti-oxidants, such as vitamins A, C, E, various members of the carotenoids, bioflavonoids and other naturally-occurring phytochemicals in food.

If the body does not have a sufficient supply of oxygen at the cellular level, the cells may ferment the glucose molecules (anaerobic) for energy rather than burn them (aerobic). Once the cells revert to this anaerobic process they no longer perform the functions they were designed for and are considered to be inefficient or unhealthy.

If the body does not get a sufficient supply of oxygen, the body will not be able to utilize nutrients efficiently. Therefore, when ATP is not sufficiently available, a less efficient (fermentation) means of creating energy occurs. This can result in even more free-radical production and less energy available to suppress these free radicals (anoxia followed by oxygenation). Remember that every action, and every process in the body, requires energy which requires a sufficient supply of oxygen!

gart in 1955, and quoted in Science, is in Appendix VII. It is invaluable information on cellular oxygen metabolism.)

Healthy cells in the body break down the carbohydrates we eat into simple "glucose" sugars. The glucose is then stored in the cells. The cells, when they need energy to perform their functions, (reproduction, heat, etc.,) take the stored glucose and in a chemical reaction with oxygen, create A. T. P. (adenosine tri-phosphate) which becomes, as described by Dr. Warburg, the "pure energy of the cell." (62, 63)

If there is a lack of oxygen at the cellular level, no life processes can take place and the cell dies. But Dr. Warburg also discovered that a poor supply of oxygen is also detrimental to the cell.

When cells lack the right amount of oxygen, the glucose in these cells begins to ferment and a chain-reaction starts taking place. Instead of living off the A.T.P., the cell begins to live off of the fermentation of the stored glucose. This reverses the cell's normal metabolic cycle.

The by-products of this fermentation process produce additional toxins which leak out into the blood stream causing additional cellular damage and taxing the immune system. The damaged cells begin to multiply, no longer functioning as they were designed and assisting the body in its various functions. These unhealthy cells (malignant or benign) drain the body of its nutritional supplies and grow in a rapid and unchecked fashion. We call groups of these cells "tumors" and the cells themselves are called "cancerous".

Here is what Dr. Warburg said in a lecture delivered in 1966 in Lindau Germany to a peer group of distinguished Nobel science recipients (the complete text is in Appendix VI):

"Summarized in a few words, the prime cause of cancer is the replacement of the respiration of oxygen in normal cells by a fermentation of sugar. All normal body cells meet their energy needs by respiration of oxygen, whereas cancer cells meet their energy needs in great part by fermentation. All normal cells are thus obligate areobes, whereas all cancer cells are partial anaerobes.

"From the standpoint of physics and the chemistry of life, this difference between normal and cancer cells is so great that one can scarcely picture a greater difference. Oxygen gas, the donor of energy in plants and animals, is dethroned in the cancer cells and replaced by an energy yielding reaction of the lowest living forms, namely, a fermentation of glucose.

"As emphasized, it is the first precondition of the proposed treatment that all growing bodies be saturated with oxygen." (62, 63)

The research by Dr. Warburg emphasizes the important point that without an adequate supply of oxygen, the body cannot function properly. Oxygen is absolutely the most important elemental nutritional

33

substance the body can possess. An abundant and consistent supply of oxygen is the basis for a healthy immune system and all bodily functions.

Thus, the lack of a consistent and quality supply of oxygen is considered by many medical experts as the root cause of all diseases that attack and destroy the body. Reduce the oxygen supply and you inhibit the production of energy, energy needed to maintain growth and the health of the body; energy needed to reduce or eliminate toxins in the body.

Chapter Four:

The Breakdown of the Immune System

"Oxygen plays a pivotal role in the proper functioning of the immune system."

Dr. Parris M. Kidd, Ph.D.
Antioxidant Adaptation

Dr. Stephen Levine and Dr. Parris M. Kidd (both well respected molecular bioligists) completed research that confirmed that "...oxygen is the source of life to all cells." (34, 37) The medical research indicates that we subject our bodies to massive amounts of physiological stress because of our poor eating and drinking habits, as well as a lack of exercise. These two factors alone rob precious oxygen from our bodies.

This situation is further complicated by the presence and increased consumption of pollutants and toxic preservatives in the water, food and the air we breathe. In fact, statistics now indicate we have over 70,000 new toxic substances to deal with than did our grandparents, and each year, we produce over 100,000,000 tons of synthetic chemicals, any one of which could seriously affect our health.

Dr. Kidd wrote: "Oxygen plays a pivotal role in the proper functioning of the immune system..." (35) especially as it relates to the system's resistance to disease, bacteria, and viruses. Dr. Levine added: "We can look at oxygen deficiency as the single greatest cause of all diseases.." (35) It is believed, and supported by a great deal of research, that a shortage of oxygen in the blood could very well be the starting point for the breakdown of the immune system.

According to Dr. Levine, "oxygen nutrition" optimizes the concentration of oxygen in relation to a natural food diet. In other words, the amount of oxygen in relation to food density is the key for excellent cell metabolism. Dr. Levine went on further to show that complex carbohydrates are oxygen rich foods. These complex carbohydrates include vegetables, whole grains, seeds, and nuts. (Fruits are too high in simple sugars to be classified as complex carbohydrates.)

As a research chemist, Dr. Levine defines a complex carbohydrate as having 16 parts of oxygen and only 14 parts carbon and hydrogen. "More than half the weight of complex carbohydrates is oxygen," he stated. "But the percentage of oxygen in fats is less than ten or at the very most fifteen percent, so fats are very low in oxygen. In fact, fats are oxygen robbers. Protein is composed of 0 to 50 percent oxygen, depending on the specific amino acid profile. It is obvious that complex carbohydrates have the most oxygen." (39)

No nutrient - whether it is protein, fatty acid, vitamin or mineral - fulfills its functions in its original form. Nutrients, as they occur in our diets, are simply mechanical substances necessary for converting the potential energy in our foods into usable chemical energy for living. For this conversion to take place, oxygen must be present.

Dr. Warburg's research adds further emphasis to these findings. He stated that sub-optimal oxygenation of tissues and cells as seen in cellular hypoxia (a lack of oxygen at the cellular level) is not only the underlying cause of diseases, like cancer, but also results in a predisposition towards degenerative diseases.

The lack of oxygen is the outstanding factor in immuno-depressive illnesses. Thus, all three researchers conclude, the increased oxygenation of the blood stream and cells will most certainly enhance and may even restore overall health.(62, 63)

Oxygen is used by the cells in many processes that break down toxic substances in the body. This process of combining a substance with oxygen at the cellular level is called "oxidation". Dr. Levine describes "oxidation" this way:

"Oxygen provides the spark of life. Nutrients provide the fuel for burning. The correct fuel/oxygen mixture is required for the best of health." (35)

A lack of oxygen in proper amounts prevents oxidation and oxygenation, two processes that energize the cells to biological regeneration. These processes are the very foundation of life and death. If the normal environment of the cell is maintained, it will not lose its growth and reproduction potential. Poor oxygen supplies will result in poor oxidation. Poor oxidation results in increased cell contamination.

Oxygen is a vital cell detoxifier. When body oxygen levels are deficient, toxins build and may eventually devastate the body functions and deplete the body of life-giving energy. Without oxygen, there can be no nourishment. Without nourishment, there can be no heat or energy and the body cannot purify itself.

A body with an excellent oxygen supply, and an unhindered development of the oxidating and oxygenation metabolic processes, will be considered healthy and sound (sound health).

Chapter Five:

Free Radicals:
Enemies Or Allies?

"When there is excessive oxidation and a deficiency of antioxidants, the excess free radicals are free to create havoc in the body. They are involved in aging, immune diseases, cancer and, of course, in chemical sensitivities and allergies"

Dr. Abram Hoffer, M.D., Ph.D.

"Minute amounts of free radicals are essential for many important functions of the immune system and other vital cellular activities."

Dr. Peter Rothschild, M.D.
Free Radicals, Stress
and Antioxidant Enzymes

Over the last 30 years, thousands of scientific studies have revealed that free radical activity represents a major cause of all degenerative diseases. These same studies also indicate, quite clearly, that there is an effective way to control and in some cases eliminate free radical damage.

Unfortunately, free radical science is totally misunderstood by the general public. Misinformation on this subject -- especially as it relates to the claim that

How Our Bodies Naturally Control Free Radicals:

A free radical is an atom or molecule missing one electron in the outer orbital shell causing the atom or molecule to carry a negative (-) electrical charge. Where two electrons should be present to insure the atom's stability, only one exists creating instability and making this atom or molecule highly reactive with other atoms or molecules in its vicinity. For this reason, free radicals are very "short-lived."

Oxygen:
The Essential Ingredient
Oxygen (O_2) is absolutely necessary for the aerobic combustion of glucose in each cell in the body.

Glucose: The Fuel
Glucose molecules in the cell are made up of carbon, hydrogen and oxygen atoms. Glucose is the "FUEL" for the cells' energy production.

A.T.P.: The Power Source
As the glucose fuel is "burned" the cells create adenosine triphosphate (ATP) the source of power for all cell, organ and body functions.

Normal Metabolism Creates Free Radicals
Creating free radicals is a naturally occurring process. During the burning of the glucose and the formation of A.T.P., free radicals are naturally

created. The body is designed to use free radicals as part of the immune system's defenses as well as diffuse and eliminate free radicals when they are not needed.

Low Oxygen = Poor Metabolism

If the body does not have a sufficient supply of oxygen at the cellular level, the cells will ferment the glucose molecules (anaerobic) for energy rather than burn them (aerobic). Once the cells revert to this anaerobic process they no longer perform the metabolic and other life functions that they were efficiently designed for. While our cells do lapse in and out of aerobic metabolism many times during the day, it is prolonged anaerobic periods that cause the greatest concern for cellular health.

Anti-oxidants:
Reducing Free Radical Life

Free radicals have a life span of typically less than 1/10,000 of a second in the blood stream. Free radical formation is typically and efficiently dampened by such anti-oxidants as vitamins A, C, E and various other food-source antioxidants.

Low cellular oxygen will prevent the body from utilizing anti-oxidants and other nutrients efficiently. Low body oxygen levels also results in greater free-radical production and less energy to suppress free radicals. Remember that every body process requires energy produced using the available oxygen in the blood stream.

oxygen is a dangerous substance to the body -- is often promoted by both the media and by manufacturers of nutrients and supplements.

What is the truth? What actually is a free radical? How and why are they created? Are all free radicals harmful to the body? Is there an effective way to deactivate or control free radicals? Finally, is oxygen the real villain that it has been made out to be? Is oxygen responsible for producing free radicals? Before we take a more in-depth look into how free radicals "react" in the body, let's look at how the experts describe these unusual molecules.

Dr. Denham Harman, M.D., Ph.D. is considered the "father" of the free radical aging theory. Currently a professor emeritus at the University of Nebraska-Omaha, Dr. Harman put forth the belief back in 1954 that unstable atoms called "free radicals" caused damage to cellular DNA that resulted in cellular death. Thus, *free radicals* were the cause of the aging process. "Chances are," wrote Dr. Harman about free radicals, that "99% are the basis for aging. Aging is the ever-increasing accumulation of changes caused or contributed to by free radicals." (15, 22)

Dr. Earl Stadtman, Chief of the Laboratory of Biochemistry of the National Heart, Lung and Blood Institute in Bethesda, M.D. concurs with Dr. Harman:

"What the human life span reflects is simply the level of free radical oxidative damage that accumulates in the cells. When enough damage accumulates, cells can't survive

42

properly anymore and they just give up."
(22)

The simplest definition of a free radical was written by Dr. Kurt Donsbach in his book *Oxygen-Oxygen-Oxygen:*

"It is an element or compound which has an unpaired or unmatched electron. This lack of balance causes the substance to have a very reactive character. However, it must be noted that these free radicals are very short-lived, usually in the one ten-thousandth of a second range. But during this short time, these free radicals can cause damage by joining with other body chemicals and changing their character, sometimes even producing a chain reaction by creating new free radicals that carry on." (19)

Dr. Peter Rothschild, in his work *Free Radicals, Stress and Antioxidant Enzymes* wrote:

"Due to their over-reactive nature, free radicals can be extremely toxic and are a direct consequence of the primary stress factors that adversely affect the immune system and threaten our health. However, this is not to imply that free radicals are always harmful or dangerous. Minute amounts of free radicals are essential for many important functions of the immune system and other vital cellular activities.

"For example, the immune system will actually generate free radicals to use in the process of removing a virus or bacteria. Only when high concentrations of free radicals are present, or when the levels of free radicals overwhelm the body's ability to remove them, does a threat to our health occur. Maintaining the balance between free radical activity and antioxidant enzyme supply is one of the important functions of the body." (55)

Free radicals are missing electrons, and in this quantum atomic state, they will do whatever they can in stealing an electron from another source. Around every atom orbit electrons in what are called shells. These shells (or sub-orbits) vary in distance from the center of the atom's nucleus.

Each sub-orbit can accommodate two electrons, each "spinning" or generating what quantum physicists call "wave forms" or "wave packets" in different directions. If one of these electrons is missing in the outer orbit the atom will seek out a matching electron. It will not stop looking for this match until it finds one. Such an unstable and reactive atom is called a free radical.

Free radicals can be of various sizes, from single atoms to more complex molecules. They can be one, two, three and four atom molecules based on oxygen, or may be formed from more complex atoms. There are many types of free radicals, but the most destructive include superoxide, hydrogen peroxide, hydroxyl, singlet oxygen (not diatomic oxygen -- O2!), polyunsaturated fatty acid radicals, organic/fatty acid hydroperoxides and oxidized proteins. (15)

It is important to point out that oxygen is not the "cause" of free radical production in the body. Oxygen doesn't cause free radicals any more than glucose causes them. However, if the body did not contain oxygen, then no oxygen free radicals could be created. This seems like a paradox, and in some ways it is.

The body produces oxygen free radicals as a natural part of metabolic energy production in each cell. As oxygen is consumed along with glucose to produce A.T.P. energy, some of the by-products of metabolism are oxygen free-radicals. The body needs energy to carry out its daily functions, like growth, maintaining body temperature, muscle action (movement) and thinking. All of these require enormous amounts of energy. Again, this energy is derived from the combustion of oxygen and glucose in power plants in each cell called the mitochondria. Like a factory that burns fuel for energy and produces smoke, the mitochondria's produces waste products which we call free radicals.

By the way, there are sources of free radicals other than those produced in the mitochondria. The free radicals from these sources may react with oxygen free radicals to cause more damage. The sources include alcohol, tobacco smoke and nicotine, industrial

45

pollution and other emissions, pesticides, pollution in water, food and the air, saturated and overheated fats, smog, radiation (including ultraviolet/U.V.), organic solvents, unprotected exposure to sunlight, detergents, paints, cleaning solvents, hair sprays, deodorants and more. It is the accumulation of these toxins that cause the greatest damage to the body. And these pollutants actually rob oxygen from the body.

Now, if the body produces free radicals as it generates energy, it only stands to reason that the body must have some mechanism to control these oxygen-free radicals as they are continuously created. If the body did not have such protection, and if, as the theory states, that oxygen free radicals can cause cellular D.N.A. damage, then without such protection the body would soon deteriorate and die. How then does the body protect itself?

The body protects itself by utilizing the electro-chemical uniqueness of antioxidants -- a group of atoms and molecules that bond with or share electrons with free radicals making these radicals stable atoms or molecules. This means that free radicals can be controlled by molecules produced in the body, like the enzymes superoxide dismutase (SOD) and gluthathione peroxidase, as well as the naturally occurring vitamins and nutrients we can daily obtain like E, C, beta-carotene and bioflavonoids. These free radical soldiers or "scavengers" deactivate free radicals.

Superoxide dismutase (SOD), produced by the body, is perhaps the most important defender against free radicals. In fact it is so important that out of over

100,000 proteins that the body produces, it is the fifth most prevalent. SOD is powerful in its ability to eliminate superoxide (O_2-) molecules! (16)

As mentioned earlier, there are both good and bad free radicals. As Joanne McAllister Smart, Managing Editor of Vegetarian Times, writes:

> "Free radicals are not all bad -- at least not if you count breathing among life's more positive experiences. Ironically, breathing is the major source of free radical production in humans. Because oxygen molecules have not one, but two unpaired electrons, the most common free radicals are built on oxygen.
>
> "All living things require energy to function. As humans we need a lot of energy to think, eat, sleep, talk and other fun things. To generate energy, cells remove electrons from sugars and add these electrons to oxygen forming highly reactive compounds. Most of these temporarily unstable molecules eventually combine with hydrogen to form stable water molecules...Free radicals are also purposely created by the immune system to fight against invading bacteria and viruses." (43)

The body *produces* free radicals as an important component of the immune system. But free radicals are supposed to cause aging, sickness and death! Do we have another paradox to deal with?

Yes! As I started out this chapter stating, oxygen is a double-edged sword. Without oxygen we die. With oxygen we subject ourselves to free-radicals as the body naturally produces energy to function and live. With oxygen we also produce the first line of defense in our immune system's battle against an invading army of pathogens which includes viruses, bacteria, yeasts and molds.

Jack Challem, a featured writer to a number of health related publications, and editor of the Nutrition Reporter, a publication that summarizes recent medical journal articles on vitamins and nutrition, explains this relationship between "the good, the bad and the ugly" this way:

"It's necessary to know that free radicals, while often the villains in what has popularly been branded as a 'biological gunfight at the OK Corral' are not always the bad guys. Free radicals are sometimes the good guys. For example, white blood cells use free radicals to destroy bacteria and virus-infected cells. According to Bruce Ames, Ph.D., of the University of California, Berkeley, these free radicals prevent immediate death from infection. In addition, with the help of other free radicals, the liver's cytochrome P-450 enzymes detoxify harmful chemicals.

"What contributes to disease and rapid aging are excessive free radicals produced by outside environmental influences. If you wipe out large numbers of good free radicals, you're handcuffing your body's immune system." (14)

Mr. Challem goes deeper into the free radical dilemma in a subsequent article he wrote for Nutrition Science News. He states that the body produces free radicals in four ways. First, most are produced as a consequence of eating and breathing. As the body produces energy some superoxide free radicals escape and can cause cellular DNA damage. (By the way, anything that increases respiration -- including exercise -- also increases free radical production!)

Second, as fatty acids are digested or broken down, hydrogen peroxide molecules are created. Some of these peroxide molecules escape and can oxidize fats in the membranes of cells thus damaging the permeability and the integrity of the membranes.

Third, enzymes produced in the liver (like cytochrome P450) are designed to detoxify the body from pollutants in water, food, air, smoke and other chemicals or toxins occurring naturally in foods. P450 thus helps prevent acute illnesses and rapid death from these poisons to the body. But as P450 and other enzymes break down these toxins, free radicals are produced that can injure healthy tissues and so contribute to aging and death.

Fourth, white blood cells -- the body's foot soldiers against invading diseases -- produce tremendous amounts of free radicals to fight infections. White blood cells "digest" bacteria and virus-infected cells and kill these pathogenic organisms with a shot-gun-like burst of free radicals (hydroxyl, superoxide, peroxide and singlet oxygen.) These same bullets can also hit and damage healthy cells. (15)

Dr. Howard Halperin at the University of Chicago adds a fifth way the body produces beneficial free radicals. He writes:

"One of life's most beautiful and dramatic moments occurs when a newborn infant takes its first breath. A baby's ability to switch quickly from its mother's circulation and take oxygen into its lungs is generated by a type of free radical." (22)

Dr. Robert Koch, discoverer of the tubercle bacillus (the cause of tuberculosis) and a staunch supporter of oxygen-based therapies, explained the purpose of free radicals in the immune system in more scientific terms:

"When its (oxygen's) activity wanes, the toxins that support pathogenic germ activity, that produce allergy, or that cause cancer, are not destroyed in the body and can execute their effects. All of these toxins depend upon their free valences between carbon atoms, between carbon and oxygen, and between carbon and nitrogen for their pathogenic action."

"Our synthetic antitoxins not only activate oxygen, but they activate the toxic free valences of germ and allergy poisons to accept the activated oxygen and thus become burned to harmless structures." (47)

Without a doubt, free radicals can do damage to the cells in our body. Recent studies indicate that free radicals bombard the cells' DNA molecules over 10,000 time a day but that severe cellular injury seldom occurs because of the body's natural antioxidant defense mechanisms. (22, 61)

In fact, according to research conducted by Dr. Bruce Ames, Director of the National Institute of Environmental Health Sciences Center at the University of California in Berkeley, these naturally produced antioxidant enzymes, vitamins, minerals and proteins race to these accident scenes and repair the damage from 99% to 99.9% of the time! (22)

Dr. Ames' research goes on the explain that the real problem is that the body simply cannot keep up with this constant repair cycle and so the result is aging. Thus, as Dr. Ames points out, the life spans of animals and humans are directly related the the body's ability to repair free radical damage. He writes:

"Normally we're OK. But it doesn't quite keep up. As you get older, more and more ... accumulates. Sunshine, for instance, is a carcinogen and 99% of its damage is repaired.

"But if you get too much sunshine, you get skin cancer and melanoma." (22)

Dr. Earl Stadtman adds:

"What the human life span reflects is simply the level of oxidative damage that accumulates in the cells...When enough damage accumulates, cells can't survive properly anymore and they just give up." (22)

It's important to mention one more time that free radicals are not left to do damage without a very efficient safety net in our bodies. This net includes the actions and reactions of groups of powerful free radical scavengers that neutralize these radicals and prevent massive cell oxidation. They accomplish this by either supplying the missing electron to a free radical or removing an extra one which stabilizes the free radical and thus stops its potential danger.

Since we know where free radicals come from and how they are created, does science also know how to reduce their effects on the body? An increasingly broad spectrum of research indicates we do indeed have part of the solution.

We cannot stop breathing -- which is a source of oxygen to keep us alive but also is a source (not the cause!) of free radicals. We can prevent the build-up of toxins and pollutants which cause the most dangerous group of free radicals which now occur in the air we breathe, water we drink and food we consume.

We can also assist the body in fighting off the aging process by making sure we have a sufficient supply of antioxidant missiles in our defensive arsenal against disease. High quality and bio-available vitamin, mineral and amino acid supplements are available from numerous companies. Fresh fruits, herbs and vegetables also supply very potent antioxidants to the body.

Free radicals are an instrumental part of the body's working mechanisms. Oxygen free radicals serve an important and critical cleansing and disinfecting purpose. Without them, sick cells, toxins and disease organisms could not be controlled or eliminated. Author and nutritionist Sonya Starr writes:

"Without the free radical oxygen, also known as O1 or nascent oxygen, 'nasty and destructive' free radicals cannot be efficiently eliminated by the body. The nascent available free radical oxygen seeks out and combines with toxic free radicals. These destructive free radicals have accumulated due to the absence of healthy 'free radical' oxygen. This absence has hindered the whole oxidative cycle of our aerobic bodies." (58)

Maharishi Ayur-Ved summarized the free radical issue in his book *Freedom from Disease: How to Control Free Radicals*:

The Body's Free-Radical Warriors:

The body uses consumed antioxidants as well as ones manufactured by the body to defend itself from the onslaught of free radicals produced as a natural part of the body's process of creating energy.

Enzymes & Proteins
superoxide dismutase (SOD)
catalase
L-glutathione
L-cysteine
gamma-linoleic acid (GLA)
co-enzyme Q10 (CoQ10)

Natural Antioxidant Sources
onions (quercetin)
black & green tea
apples
carrots
garlic (allicin)
bilberry
turmeric
oregano
mint
rosemary
summer savory
thyme
dill
barley grass

broccoli
brussels sprouts
cabbage
wheat germ
shiitake mush-rooms
flax ssed oil
sesame oil
caraway oil
echinacea root
acidophilus

Vitamins & Minerals
zinc
selenium
manganese
copper
chromium
Vitamin A
Vitamin C
Vitamin E
bioflavonoids
beta-carotene
pycnogenol
kaempferol
myricetin
Apigenin
leuteolin

"They are an inescapable feature of all oxygen based life. As part of the life-giving process that creates energy in every cell, free radicals are created as toxic waste. When the immune systems sends special forces to fight infection, free radicals are used as a weapon...If the body takes in pesticides, industrial chemicals, processed foods, cigarette smoke, or alcohol, free radicals are the most common result. And when the mind and body come under stress, free radicals are mass produced." (3)

Lastly, many researchers would have us believe that less oxygen in the body would result in less free radical production. Therefore, they would further clarify, taking oxygen supplementation would be actually harmful to the body since any increase in oxygen would relate to an increase in free radical production. But some logical assumptions are not necessarily true, as in this case.

Research conducted for the U.S. Army's Environmental Medicine Research Institute by Dr. Wayne Askew, Ph.D., now the Director of the Division of Foods and Nutrition at the University of Utah, indicates a different oxygen story. Studying oxidative stress and the need for antioxidants at high altitudes, Dr. Askew determined that less oxygen increased oxidative stress and the need for additional antioxidant supplementation to deal with that stress. (2) To put it in another way, less oxygen to the body increases the production of free radicals as well as our need for a greater supply of antioxidants to neutralize the free radicals.

Dr. Askew's findings agree with the theories proposed by Dr. Robert Koch some 60 years earlier:

"When adequate molecular oxygen is available, protection against disease is provided. When molecular oxygen is not available, the free radicals formed by the dehydrogenation cannot combine oxygen and forms a peroxide-free radical to continue the combustion process.

"The free radical can do only one thing: add to the closest double bond at hand. This is the same double bond that activates the carbonyl group which removed its hydrogen atom to form the free radical. By this action, the host cell's energy production mechanism is paralyzed by the integration of the foreign substance of fuel product. Normal function is blocked and can be forced beyond physiological control by the input of vicarious energy, which can result in multiple allergies and / or cancer." (47)

(See Appendix IV for an in-depth explanation about free radicals.)

Chapter Six:

Pain Is Caused
By A Lack Of Oxygen

"Insufficient oxygen means insufficient biological energy that can result in anything from mild fatigue to life threatening disease. The link between insufficient oxygen and disease has now been firmly established."

*Dr. Spencer Way, M.D.
Journal of the American
Association of Physicians*

The traditional definition of pain is any unpleasant sensation occurring in varying degrees of severity as a consequence of injury, disease, or emotional disorder causing suffering. There is a growing body of scientific evidence that indicates that the reduction of cellular oxygen can affect the body in such a manner that the result is an increase in pain as muscles, organs and body systems no longer function properly.

Dr. C. Samuel West, a specialist in the science of lymphology and a distinguished member of the international Society of Lymphology, has proven that food present in cells without enough oxygen will turn into waste products (like lactic acid) and fat. He has written that the less oxygen present in the cells, the more pain we experience. (64)

Dr. West is a strong advocate of exercise since a lack of exercise reduces circulation and thus the transfer of oxygen to the cells. This leads to high blood pressure and fluid retention. There are a number of factors that prevent aerobic metabolism and favor anaerobic metabolism: a lack of A.D.P. to accept phosphate to form A.T.P.; a lack of NAD+ to accept hydrogen to form NADN; a lack of oxygen at the cellular level caused by physiological conditions that prevent an adequate supply of oxygen in the blood stream.

Any one of these conditions will upset the metabolic processes and functioning of the cell. These cells, lacking sufficient oxygen, start manufacturing improper chemicals and soon these cells and their surrounding cells become weak and unhealthy. If prolonged, the organs as well as the entire immune system may start breaking down and malfunctioning providing conditions which may allow disease organisms to flourish.

A lack of cellular A.T.P. drastically alters the body's sodium-potassium balance in the individual cells, in the blood stream, and in the fluid that surrounds the cells. The chemical change also alters and reduces the "electrical fields" in the cells, and the blood stream. Once this electrical change occurs, minerals begin to "fall out" of the fluids surrounding the cells and the bloodstream, and start sticking together in what is called "mineral deposits". If these minerals settle in the joints, arthritis occurs; in the eyes, cataracts occur. When they settle in the arteries, we describe the process as "hardening of the arteries."

Our muscles also respond to electrical charges sent by the brain. These messages tell the muscles to contract and release. Anything that upsets this delicate and intricate electrical transfer of energy, as does a lack of adequate amounts of A.T.P., will cause the muscles to spasm and work or respond poorly causing discomfort and even extreme levels of pain.

Prolonged or excessive stress to the muscles, joints or organs in the body will cause the body to increase the production of specific hormones designed to relieve the body of pain. (These hormones can include cortisol and epinephrine (which we call adrenaline.) These same hormones, however, cause dramatic changes in metabolism, blood pressure and heart rates.

As the pressure, stress, anxiety or prolonged physical activities increase, these blood hormones become trapped in the tissues. As Dr. Kurt Donsbach, N.D. explains:

"These blood proteins attract and retain water in the body tissue, creating a localized edema thus bringing about swelling. The edema will in turn slow down the the distribution of oxygen and the disposal of carbon dioxide from the cells. The lack of oxygen, the chemicals released from damaged cells, and the pressure to the nerve endings, will create pain.

"Tissue that is inflamed tends to lose flexibility and thus creates an initial stiffness. The stiffness, accumulation of blood proteins, fluids and salts, and the transformation of energy into heat, will precipitate and crystallize substances like calcium and uric acid creating a vicious cycle that culminates with chronic pain and deformities." (18)

Chapter Seven:

Our Diet Determines the Availability of Oxygen

"Rubble, garbage, toxins, refuse, debris and anything useless are destroyed by oxygen and carried out of the system. Just as a clean house holds little interest to passing flies, likewise an oxygen rich body is a difficult fortress to assail."

Brian Goulet, Certified Herbalist
Canadian Journal of
Health and Nutrition

We live in the world of fast-foods and instant-gratification. In addition, no modern society consumes more red meats and dairy products than does America. Research currently estimates that over 45% of the American diet is fat. Unfortunately, animal and dairy products contain high concentrations of cholesterol.

While the body needs some "good" cholesterol to run efficiently, (like those from grains or nuts,) the cholesterol from meats and dairy products passes directly in to the blood stream and begins to "trap" blood proteins which are so important for stabilizing and regulating the flow of oxygen to the cells.

Excessive consumption of cholesterol/fat-ridden food robs oxygen from the blood stream. Fats easily combine with oxygen and form "free radicals". These free radicals use more oxygen to form peroxides that damage and destroy the cells.

As far back as 1977, it was reported in the Scientific American (February Issue) that "...cholesterol epoxide (peroxide) and other substances formed from cholesterol will cause cells to mutate and which will cause cancer." (44) This is how fatty foods, which are consumed by so many Americans, cause an oxygen deficiency which provides physiological conditions that can increase the onset of cancer in those with a propensity for such a disease.

Cells that lose their ability to utilize oxygen can become cancerous. (*See Dr. Warburg's lecture notes in Appendix VI for more detailed information on the relationship of cancer and low oxygen levels.*) These cells have been oxygen-starved for so long that they undergo a metabolic "shift" and revert to a metabolism that does not use oxygen as the spark for cellular respiration (called anaerobic metabolism).

This is, of course, the ultimate and last state of cellular degeneration which is caused by a low oxygen life-style. It is also interesting that research shows that people who consume very high quantities of fat have a far greater incidence of cancer as well as other degenerative diseases.

Thus, cholesterol rich foods, (those lacking the life-giving oxygen found in raw vegetables, et., which are easily converted into energy,) are converted into toxic waste and fat in the cells. This toxic waste and fat in the cells impedes the nutrient supply to the cells from the blood stream. In addition, all the current nutritional research clearly indicates that foods high in sugars, salts, fats and cholesterol are directly responsible for problems like kidney and heart diseases, liver damage, high blood pressure, hardening of the arteries, obesity, and strokes.

Dr. Levine has described the consequences of cellular oxygen deficiencies in this way: it is ...

"An acidic condition, caused by the the accumulation of acidic by-products, occurs in poorly oxygenated cells. Soft drinks, caffeine, alcohol, and red meats are among the substances that cause systemic (whole body) acidity where there is an excess of positively charged hydrogen ions (H+)." (39)

When excessive numbers of hydrogen ions are in the tissue environment they will combine with (and thus utilize) oxygen resulting in an oxygen deficiency state.

"When cells are deprived of oxygen, lactic acid accumulates and the cellular environment becomes acidic. This reduces available oxygen for the primary function of metabolism because more oxygen is needed to neutralize the acid." (39)

Meat and dairy foods, which are high in cholesterol, break down (dissolve) in our stomach and intestines. These foods are potentially harmful if consumed in excess since their chemical by-products may cause deterioration, pain and disease. These by-products dilate (widen or expand) the capillaries making the distance that the water has to travel to and from the cells much greater.

The greater the distance that the fluids must travel, in the same amount of time, the less the transfer of nutrients, oxygen and minerals. Also the less toxins, waste products, poisons, etc. are transferred back out of the cells and in to the blood stream. The waste products, toxins, etc., start to accumulate in the cells.

Stretched capillary walls allow the blood proteins to escape and lodge themselves between the cells. The trapped proteins permit the accumulation of excess fluids around the cells. This prevents the cells from getting the very oxygen they need and so the glucose begins to ferment resulting in electrical changes as the mineral and salt balances change as well.

Oxygen rich red blood cells carry a negative electrical charge. They travel through the capillaries single file. As the capillaries dilate, and the electrical balance of our body changes because of a lack of oxygen, these blood cells are now dispersed over a greater volume in the capillaries and are unable to travel the now greater distances to the cells.

To further complicate matters, the red blood cells, because of the electrical change, begin to clump together to cause a microscopic traffic jam in the capillaries. This further dilates the capillary pores and allows more blood proteins to escape and lodge in the spaces around the cells. This produces more fluid around the cells and the process repeats itself until the cells begin to die because of lack of oxygen.

Those suffering from physiological conditions (ailments) as a direct result of diets high in fat intake have also seriously affected the immune system's ability to compensate for the increased amounts of toxins in the blood stream. Increased levels of toxins create conditions (both chemical as well as a lack of oxygen) where pathogenic micro-organisms can thrive. These micro-organisms also spew out additional toxic wastes for the body's organs to metabolize and eliminate to prevent the poisoning of the cells.

Because fats and toxins rob oxygen from the body, the body's oxygen levels continue to decline. As the levels decline, cellular respiration, which requires oxygen, becomes less efficient and more waste products and toxins accumulate both inside and outside the cells. Soon, as the body attempts to adapt to these low oxygen levels to survive, the entire body is so deprived of oxygen that only the most vital organic functions get the available oxygen, with the brain and heart muscles receiving the lion's share.

This extreme oxygen-deprived condition is called hypoxemia and the result of prolonged low tissue oxygenation is tissue damage and even cell death. Patricia A. McGaffigan, R.N., M.S., identified five major causes of hypoxemia in her article "Hazards of Hypoxemia". (44)

(1) Contrary to many medical professionals beliefs, only low levels of "inspired" oxygen are available to individuals at very high altitudes. While the body does adapt itself to this change in atmospheric pressure, the fact is that less oxygen is consumed reducing the effectiveness of the body's respiratory and metabolic functioning. Prolonged high-altitude conditions, like those experienced by mountain climbers, can result in temporary brain damage and even death.

(2) Conditions which prevent full lung ventilation can affect the body's ability to reach optimum blood oxygen saturation. These conditions can include neurological diseases, the effect of narcotics on the nervous and musculature system, musculoskeletal disorders that prevent the proper functioning of the respiratory muscles, respiratory obstructions or scar tissue damage to the lungs as a result of diseases like chronic bronchitis, pneumonia, asthma, smoking or other toxic fumes or gasses which damage the alveoli in the lungs.

(3) The membranes which permit the passing of oxygen and carbon dioxide between the capillaries and the alveoli may become thicker. This can be caused by diseases like chronic bronchitis, pneumonia, asthma, fibrosis, pulmonary edema, smoking or other toxic fumes or gasses.

(4) Poor pulmonary circulation can and does reduce oxygen distribution in the body. This occurs because of a variety of disorders including damaged capillaries and arterial plaque build-up.

Oxygenating the Red Blood Cell

Each erythrocyte (red blood cell) contains over 300 million hemoglobin molecules, and each molecule can bind four molecules of diatomic oxygen (O2).

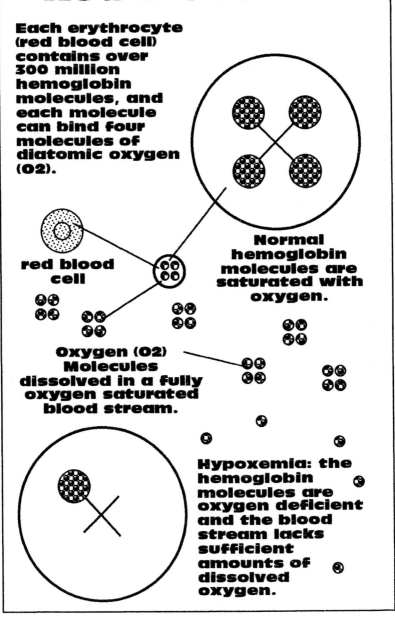

red blood cell

Normal hemoglobin molecules are saturated with oxygen.

Oxygen (O2) Molecules dissolved in a fully oxygen saturated blood stream.

Hypoxemia: the hemoglobin molecules are oxygen deficient and the blood stream lacks sufficient amounts of dissolved oxygen.

(5) Lower blood oxygen levels can be the result of anemia disorders, sleep apnea, those suffering from upper abdominal or thoracic pain resulting in shallow breathing and carbon monoxide poisoning.

While Ms. McGaffigan points out that some of the causes of hypoxemia are medical or genetic abnormalities, many of the causes are dietary related. Poor nutrition is at the heart of most degenerative problems that prevent the uptake and utilization of life giving oxygen. Certainly an improved diet and regular exercise will enhance overall health and oxygenation and must not be overlooked nor minimized. However, supplemental oxygen (oxygen therapies) can also help in bringing the body back to its normal, healthy state. As Ms. McGaffigan confirms:

> "You can administer supplemental oxygen by various methods and at different doses depending on the patient's degree of hypoxemia." (44)

Dr. Stephen Levine, Ph.D. summarized the conditions leading to a condition of hypoxemia in this manner:

> "In all serious disease states, we find a concomitant low oxygen state. Low oxygen in the body is a sure indicator for disease. Hypoxemia, or lack of oxygen in the tissues, is the fundamental cause of all degenerative disease." (39)

Chapter Eight:

Drugs, Disease & the Immune System

"The link between insufficient oxygen and disease has now been firmly established."

Dr. W. Spencer Way
Journal of the American Association of Physicians

Most individuals when they become "sick" turn to conventional medicine to correct the problem. Conventional approaches include prescription drugs, over-the-counter drugs, radiation and chemical (chemo) therapies, and surgery.

Researchers have learned, however, that many traditional cures for illnesses have side-effects. Antibiotics, for example, are effective for removing many pathogenic bacteria from the body. Many lives have been saved by using penicillin as well as other antibiotics in combating bacterial infections.

Unfortunately, traditional antibiotic approaches are no longer as effective as they once were. Many bacteria are becoming resistant to our past arsenal of drug ammunition. As fast as pharmaceutical companies come up with new drugs to fight new strains of these organisms, the strains mutate, change their cellular and metabolic structures, (bacteria transfer genes among themselves increasing their resistance to specialized drugs!), become stronger, more resilient and so present a new dreadful challenge to the medical community. Current information indicates that of the over 100 antibiotics in existence today, there is at least one strain of micro-organism that resists one or more of these wonder drugs.

More and more research is pointing to the proliferation and easy access to prescription drugs (antibiotics) and the repeated and the extensive use of these antibiotics as the single most significant factor in the mutation of micro-organisms. The World Health Organization (W.H.O.) reported that over 4.3 million people died in 1990 alone of respiratory infections, primarily from pneumonia.

The New England Journal of Medicine reported a new outbreak of whooping cough in 1993. In 1994, Time Magazine reported a resistant cholera epidemic that killed over 50,000 people in Rawanda. (65, 66, 67)

There are other infectious diseases that are resisting current prescription drugs. Lyme disease has stricken at least 50,000 Americans since it was discovered in 1976. A Bengal cholera strain killed over 5,000 people in Bangladesh in 1996 not to mention tens of thousands that became seriously ill. E. coli O157 is a new food bacteria that killed two and sickened over 500 people who ate at Jack-in-the-Box Restaurants in the U.S. during 1996. In Japan, the same bacteria sickened over 10,000 people. It has now become the leading cause of kidney failure in children today. (65, 66, 67)

The Rise of the Super Bugs!

Just a few emerging drug-resistant infectious diseases that worry most scientists today:

◆**Lyme Disease:** a tick-born disease that causes chronic arthritis and heart problems. At least 50,000 Americans have been stricken since it was discovered in 1976.

◆**Hantavirus:** a virus carried by rodents originally from Southeast Asia but now present in the U.S. Southwest where it has killed at least 18 people since late May of 1996.

◆**E-coli O157:** a new food bacteria that killed 2 and sickened over 500 in the U.S., infected over 10,000 in Japan in 1996 and is the leading cause of kidney failure in children today.

◆**Filovirus:** a baffling flesh-eating virus emanating from Africa that has devastated towns in Zaire and Sudan. The Zaire strain, called Ebola, has an 80% mortality rate and was considered the most lethal virus until AIDS.

◆**Streptococcal bacteria:** a new Group A strep strain was the one that killed puppeteer Jim Henson. It is a fast-killing bacteria that resembles toxic shock syndrome. It is believed to have come to the U.S. from Scandanavia. Doctors are still baffled by it and there is no cure.

Here is but one common example from a recent Associated Press news release which explains the challenges facing medical practitioners today:

"A staph germ that causes thousands of often deadly infections among hospital patients each year is becoming resistant to medicine's drug of last resort and could soon prove unstoppable. A new strain of stapholococcus areus bacteria that was discovered in a Japanese infant showed resistance for the first time against vancomycin, which has been around since 1970 and is used when other antibiotics fail.

"...Doctors have long known that many common bacteria are growing resistant to antibiotics. The resistance is attributed to the overuse of antibiotics and the failure of some patients to take their medicine properly.

"Penicillin was a wonder drug that killed staph germs when it became available in 1947. Within a decade, some strains grew resistant. Then came methicillin in the 1960s, then vancomycin, which was so potent it was regarded as medicine's 'silver bullet' against staph.

"'We have been living since 1970 using vancomycin with no fear that any staph was going to be resistant to it' said Dr. Robert Haley, chief of epidemiology at University of Texas Southwestern Medical Center in Dallas and former chief of C.D.C.'s (Center for Disease Control) hospital infections branch. This changes the whole game.'" (65)

Each week more examples are appearing in dozens of major publications indicating clearly that both the medical profession and the pharmaceutical companies are losing the battle against disease. This again is contrary to the belief that we are eradicating disease from modern society. To quote a recent article in the Science/Environment section in a regional newspaper:

"When antibiotics hit the market in the 1950s, doctors jubilantly predicted an end to infectious diseases -- and by the 1980s, half of all drug companies had stopped developing antibiotics, believing the battle won. But the bugs fought back. Today, many bacteria are impervious to medicine...More than 13,000 Americans are dying each year from drug resistant bacteria -- and doctors warn the problem is steadily worsening." (65)

In addition to the increased personal use of antibiotics, more studies are indicating that the use of antibiotics by farmers in animal feed is also compounding the problem of mutating microbes. Livestock ranchers use antibiotics to prevent diseases in animals as well as promote animal growth. These chemicals remain in the tissues and organs of animals used for meat food and when they are consumed by humans the levels of drugs in each of our bodies increases dramatically. In addition, milk products contain even more drugs used to enhance the growth as well as the milk production of cows and are used to minimize bovine diseases. All take their toll on our bodies, especially the immune system.

As these toxins and drugs combine in our bodies, this new chemical "soup" provides an environment that is perfect for the proliferation of pathogenic organisms. The body must use its precious oxygen supply to convert these toxins into less harmful substances. At the same time, the immune system will work overtime, consuming oxygen as one if its primary defense mechanisms to fight off the growth of bacteria, viruses, yeasts and other organisms that thrive in such an environment. Because this soup contains antibiotics, only the strongest, most resilient and resistant strains will survive making the final condition of the body far worse than it was in the beginning.

In a recent article in the popular ""People" magazine (November 9, 1998), titled "Bad Bad Bugs", the magazine reflects the growing concern of Dr. Mitchell Cohen, Director of the Division of Bacterial and Mycotic Diseases of the National Center for Infectious Disease of the Centers for Disease Control and Prevention in Atlanta, Georgia. The article begins:

"In time, improper handling of antibiotics and natural evolution conspired to allow bacteria to adapt in order to defend themselves against antibiotics. 'Bacteria have a tremendous evolutionary advantage,' says Cohen. 'They reproduce a lot quicker than we do, and there are a lot more of them.' As a result, bacterial diseases thought to be virtually dormant, such as tuberculosis, meningitis and salmonella, have reappeared in recent years in new drug-resistant forms. Viral diseases, such as various flu strains, HIV and the newly discovered and potentially deadly hepatitis C, are resistant to antibiotics and also pose new challenges to researchers."

The overuse and misuse of antibiotics brings back memories of the earlier part of the 1900s when contracting an infectious disease was like receiving a death sentence.

"It's not that too many antibiotics have led us astray," says Dr. Jeffrey Fisher, M.D., author of *The Plague Makers* (Simon & Schuster). It's the inappropriate use of antibiotics that has brought on the dangerous propagation of resistant strains of bacteria. This isn't a new phenomenon. It's existed since the early '40s when penicillin first came on the market." (65)

A number of current studies indicate that the recent drastic increase in Candida albicans yeast infections is primarily due to the widespread use of antibiotics and the resulting decline in available body oxygen. Candida, a pathogenic yeast problem primarily affecting the urinary tracts of women, has become resistant to most antibiotics and now infects many of the body's internal organs (systemic infection) of both men and women. Dr. Stephen Levine wrote:

"Hypoxia in the patient is a major contributing factor to yeast susceptibility...Adequate cellular oxygenation is therefore critical to cell-mediated immunity...However, the single most important substance for life -- oxygen -- may be the most powerful immune-stimulant of all." (39)

Another concern of medical professionals is that many antibiotics may also remove beneficial as well as pathogenic bacteria. This situation creates an imbalance which could lead to an overgrowth of Candida as well as many other detrimental organisms. Therefore, when we use antibiotics, we make a trade-off.

We often sacrifice our beneficial bacteria to rid ourselves of the pathogenic bacteria. While antibiotics have importance in life-threatening situations, to use them routinely for every ill is considered by many practitioners to be inappropriate and could even be dangerous to our health.

When the body encounters pathogens, (like viruses, fungi, bacteria, etc.,) in the blood stream or in tissues, the immune system's white blood cells will surround or "engulf" these invaders. They then bombard these pathogens with self-generated free-radicals which scientists call "superoxides." These "superoxides" are manufactured in the white blood cells during normal cellular metabolism using the oxygen they get from the blood stream.

If the immune system is working properly, it will generate more anti-oxidant enzymes to remove the free-radicals to protect the surrounding tissues. The importance of this anti-oxidant defense system cannot be overstated. Without it, the immune system actually works against the body by generating too many free-radicals which will go about doing damage to the surrounding tissue and our bodies. Although there are other factors, this breakdown in the immune system in many people has helped create an epidemic of auto-immune diseases like lupus and rheumatoid arthritis.

Dr. Hans Kugler, Ph.D. is a noted research scientist that has monitored the critical link between toxins and compromised immune system functions. He reported in *Preventative Medicine Update* (32) that over the last 40 years our immune systems have declined in their effectiveness against disease by more than 50%. He also points out that toxic chemicals damage our reproductive organs especially pesticides used on fruits and vegetables. These chemicals are "hormone disrupters" that mimic female estrogen and block the production of testosterone. Dr. Kugler describes this as

"...the interaction between a handicapped immune system and the rise in many cancers, the sudden appearance of new and previously unknown diseases -- and most likely -- other diseases that are immune related." (32)

If the over-use and misuse of antibiotics has been one of the chief causes for the breakdown of the immune system's ability to fight off disease, can increasing the oxygen level of the blood stream really improve the functioning of the immune system?

Chapter Nine:

Preventative Alternative Therapies: Re-charging the Immune System

"If deficiencies of less vital elements such as vitamins, minerals and enzymes can rob the human body of its health and vitality, how much more damage must result from a deficiency of oxygen, the element universally acknowledged to be the most vital to life?"

The Townsend Letter for Doctors

Oxygen is both a life-giver as well as a "killer." It is one of the body's primary guardians and protectors against unfriendly bacteria and other disease organisms. In fact, one of oxygen's major functions is the "disintegration" of pathogenic organisms in a process called oxidation.

Oxidation is a process where electrons are exchanged between oxygen and another molecule or element creating a new molecule. During this "exchange" process the donating element or molecule is changed either in its structure or its function while the oxygen atom retains its integrity. The simplest example of oxidation is the conversion of iron in air to

How Oxygen Atoms Destroy Invading Pathogens

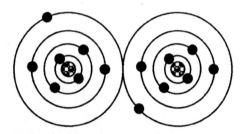

Two singlet oxygen atoms sharing electrons to form a stable diatomic oxygen (O2) molecule.

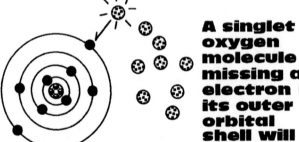

A singlet oxygen molecule missing an electron in its outer orbital shell will seek stability by acquiring an electron from a donor, in this case an electron from an anaerobic bacteria. During the exchange, the bacteria's cellular structural integrity is breached and the cell's metabolic processes are destroyed.

rust (iron oxide). Apples that have been cut into slices will turn brown because of oxidation.

Oxygen atoms are intrinsically in need of a single electron to become fully stable. Every atom is surrounded by orbiting pairs of electrons which give the atom its stability, its electrical charge ("positive" if it has extra orbiting electrons and "negative" if it is missing electrons,) and which determine the atom's ability to combine with other atoms to form more complex molecules. The strength of the attraction between atoms determines the stability of the molecules that have been created by two or more atoms.

Some molecules are quite strong and resist disintegration. Others are relatively weak and break apart easily into their component atomic parts. Hydrogen peroxide, for example, is the combination of two hydrogen atoms and two oxygen atoms (H_2O_2).

In the presence of heat, sunlight (ultraviolet rays,) or when in the presence of anything acidic, hydrogen peroxide's atoms break apart to release a singlet oxygen atom (O_1) leaving the three remaining atoms to form the very strong and stable water molecule (H_2O). The singlet oxygen atom is highly unstable and needs a electron to reach a stable state. It is in this state that this single molecule will grab electrons from any other atom or molecule in its vicinity. Luckily for us, anaerobic (non-air/oxygen tolerant) unicellular bacteria, yeasts, parasites, viruses, molds, and fungi become the perfect electron donors.

The body contains both beneficial as well as harmful microbes. Beneficial microbes like the ones that inhabit the intestinal tract and aid in the digestive process, like acidophilus and beneficial E-coli, thrive in an oxygen-rich environment. These organisms are called "aerobic" or air-tolerant. However, non-beneficial (pathogenic) organisms can only exist and can only reproduce in a reduced or non-oxygen environment. These organisms are called "anaerobic" or non-air tolerant.

The current research clearly indicates that, regardless of the genetic make-up of an anaerobic organisms, whenever these microbes are subjected to the presence of oxygen, these organisms self-destruct. One of the more technical explanations of oxygen's "mode of action" is that oxygen, (in its various configurations, i.e. O1, O2, O3 , etc.,) interferes and disrupts a pathogenic organism's cytoplasmic membrane.

Oxygen's oxidizing action appears to prevent the uptake of amino acids while at the same time disorganizing this membrane. This action creates a tear in the membrane structure which allows the organism's low molecular weight cellular contents to leak out. It is this cellular cytoplasmic breach that actually destroys the organism.

Oxygen, therefore, is naturally selective in what it kills. Unlike drugs and antibiotics which may and usually kill all bacteria in the body, oxygen kills only harmful bacteria while allowing beneficial bacteria to thrive thus insuring good health.

In addition, as we've previously discussed, oxygen is the key ingredient to healthy cellular metabolism. What one element is as versatile and crucial to our existence than oxygen? Oxygen truly is, as Dr. Stephen Levine stated, "the spark of life." (39)

Given oxygen's powerful restorative and anti-microbial properties, it can come as no surprise that a number of therapeutic protocols and theories have been developed by both the traditional medical and alternative medical professions. Space does not permit an in-depth study of the history and the diversity of alternative oxygen therapies available today. (A Brief outline of the first 150 years of oxygen therapy research may be found in Appendix IX.) For those with an appetite for detail, I do recommend the well documented book by journalist Ed McCabe called *O2xygen Therapies: A New Way of Approaching Disease* (42) or the short book by Dr. Kurt Donsbach called *Oxygen - Oxygen - Oxygen.* (19)

In general, the term "oxygen therapies" refers to any process that increases the available oxygen in the blood stream or any regimen that enhances the body's ability to utilize, retain or promote oxygen absorption. These therapies can be as simple as breathing exercises to more complex nutritional and therapeutic approaches developed and used successfully over the last 50 or so years.

Nathaniel Altman, author of the book Oxygen Healing Therapies, presents this definition of oxygen therapy and how the therapy works:

> "Oxygen therapies enhance the body's immune system and are therefore used in treating a great variety of illnesses. More than fif-

ty diseases have been treated with oxygen therapy by doctors in the U.S. including candida, cancer, dermatitis, gynecological infections, diabetes, HIV-related problems, asthma and the Epstein-Barr virus.

"The effects of oxygen therapies are two-fold. First, they increase the level of oxygen compounds used by the immune system to fight illness. These compounds are biochemically reactive free radicals which, in low doses, can safely eliminate harmful bacteria, viruses, yeasts and parasites. Second, oxygen therapies increase the delivery of oxygen to the cells and therefore promote cellular respiration, which is fundamental to all life processes." (1)

Here are just a few of the more accepted oxygen therapies:

Breathing or Inhalation Therapies: breathing exercises are designed to utilize a greater amount of lung surface area to transfer more oxygen to the blood stream and to remove more carbon dioxide from the blood stream. It is believed that the average person uses only about 50% of the lungs' capacity. Therefore, deeper breathing exercises should theoretically increase blood oxygen saturation.

For those with more serious bronchial or respiratory problems, bottled oxygen therapies may be prescribed by a medical practitioner. Pure 100% oxygen gas is very toxic to the lungs because of its oxidation potential. Therefore oxygen administered using this therapy is usually no more than 20% of the air inside a container which approximates the oxygen content in normal air.

Nutritional Therapies: research has shown that a number of vitamins, minerals, amino acids and enzymes play an important role in the creation of and use of oxygen in the body's normal metabolic cycle. One of the body's most important and abundant enzymes is superoxide dismutase (S.O.D.) and is found in every cell in the body.

S.O.D. fights harmful free radicals and turns them, along with the enzyme catalase, into stable oxygen and hydrogen peroxide and then finally into oxygen and water. Low levels of S.O.D. increase free radical damage to the body and decrease oxygen availability.

Co-enzyme Q10 (CoQ10) is found in every cell and is essential in the transfer of electrons from one atom or one molecule to another. The human body will not function without an adequate supply of CoQ10. This enzyme has been described as the "spark" that ignites the oxygen in the cells which in turn react with glucose to create A.T.P. fuel energy. Thus CoQ10 regulates the oxygen supply to the mitochondria to increase or decrease oxygen as required by the cells and the body.

Germanium is a trace mineral that is crucial for balancing the oxygen content of the cells and helping to regulate the cell's bio-electricity. Germanium, in regulating oxygen levels, enhances the immune system. This mineral also helps remove toxic minerals from the body including mercury, cadmium and lead.

Iron is the most important mineral that helps regulate, when combined in the red blood cells' hemoglobin molecule, as well as transport oxygen to every cell in the body. A lack of iron (anemia) results in poor body oxygen and an increase in a number of diseases. Women are particularly subject to iron deficiencies.

Ginseng is a root that has been used for over 4,000 years to help build endurance and alertness. Recently, research has indicated that ginseng contains high amounts of oxygen. In addition, studies indicate that ginseng helps increase oxygen levels in the blood as well as enhance pulmonary (breathing) activity.

Ginkgo biloba is an ancient, long-living tree whose leaves yield flavonglycosides which are powerful free-radical scavengers and tissue/cell membrane stabilizers. Ginkgo strengthens and improves circulation thus potentially increasing the oxygen circulation as well.

Ginger is another botanical that promotes blood and oxygen circulation while also providing over 12 natural anti-oxidants more powerful than vitamin E. Ginger also helps increase the body's absorption of other nutrients.

Magnesium peroxide is a remarkable mineral oxide that delivers substantial amounts of oxygen when potentiated by stomach acid or citric acid. As far back as 1929 formulations containing magnesium peroxide were used as a therapy and promoted by Dr. F.M. Eugene Blass considered to be one of the "fathers" of oxygen therapies. His products, called Magozone, Calzone, Malcazone and Homozone, have been used to deliver cleansing and healing oxygen to countless individuals all over the world.

Hydrogen Peroxide Therapies: over 5,000 articles have been published in the medical journals about hydrogen peroxide during the last 50 years. Most discuss the disinfecting and apparent healing properties of this remarkable molecule that easily breaks down into water and oxygen. It is the release of the singlet oxygen atom (O1) that provides so much benefit to the body.

Hydrogen peroxide is manufactured by the body as an instrumental part of the body's first line of defense against invading pathogens. The release of the oxygen atom -- which occurs when hydrogen peroxide meets a pathogen in the blood stream -- deactivates the cellular integrity of that pathogen. (See Appendix IX for more in depth information about hydrogen peroxide therapies.)

The manufacturing or "creation" of hydrogen peroxide is the function of the white blood cells. However, the body acquires hydrogen peroxide in a number of healthy foods including fruits and some vegetables. Hydrogen peroxide is also a key ingredient in colostrum, the first milk that babies drink from their mothers' breasts. (See Appendix IV on Colostrum.)

Traditional hydrogen peroxide therapies include the consumption of diluted food grade hydrogen peroxide, interveinous drips and injections of the highly diluted solution.

Ozone Therapies: Ozone is a gas molecule containing three oxygen atoms (O_3) joined together in a weak electrical bond. It is present in the atmosphere, and its blue color is what gives the sky its wonderful blue hues.

The ozone molecule is relatively unstable. It quickly breaks apart into a diatomic oxygen molecule (O_2) and a singlet oxygen molecule (O_1) in approximately 30 -40 minutes.

As far back as 1785, early scientists noted ozone's distinctive odor and disinfecting properties. It was not until 1840 that ozone got its "name" from the Greek "ozein" which means "odorant".

Ozone has not only been used as treatment for many wounds, it is now used extensively to purify water in residential and commercial pools and in waste water treatment plants around the world. Because ozone breaks down into harmless oxygen molecules, it is the ideal replacement for carcinogenic chlorine in these applications.

Ozone has been used as a blood treatment to kill viruses and to increase blood oxygenation. Studies of ozone "blown" over wounds show a dramatic improvement in the healing of those wounds as well as a significant reduction in infections. Burns particularly respond well to ozone treatments.

Ozone is 10 times more soluble in water than atmospheric oxygen (O_2) and has been bubbled in bath water to help treat and disinfect the skin for eczema and skin ulcers. It can also be added to drinking water to help increase blood oxygen levels, though the water needs to be immediately consumed since ozone decomposes so quickly into its oxygen parts.

Ozone does have several drawbacks. The singlet oxygen molecule is highly reactive oxidative atom. If not used or administered properly, ozone can cause "burns" to the skin or organs. If inhaled in large quantities, ozone can also be toxic. Ozone should never be administered for any alternative therapy situation unless under the supervision of a medical practitioner.

Hyperbaric Oxygen Therapies: For many decades, hyperbaric oxygen (HBO) chambers were used to treat decompression sickness and air embolisms of divers or aviators. During the early 1960s, HBO was proposed as a treatment for cancer, heart attacks, senility and other conditions though the medical profession, as a whole, discounted its use and benefits.

HBO therapy involves the inhalation of oxygen rich air under a pressure greater than one atmosphere. This increased atmospheric pressure helps deliver more oxygen to the tissues and cells to enhance healing as well as to improve the immune system's ability to fight off infection.

Medical research indicates that HBO therapy provides varying benefits for decompression sickness, carbon monoxide poisoning, acute tissue damage and bacterial and viral infections. Reports indicate that the Ebola (flesh eating) virus was controlled in a number of victims that were fortunate enough to undergo HBO treatments.

Despite over a century of use in medical settings, HBO still remains a controversial therapy among the medical community today. Still, in spite of the controversey, more and more HBO centers are opening up in cities all across America and throughout Europe.

Stabilized Oxygen Therapies: the last 25 years have seen the introduction of a new generation of oxygen therapy alternatives that can be safely and effectively self-administered. These stabilized oxygen (SO) therapies primarily involve the consumption of solutions containing oxygen salts or dissolved oxygen. The next chapter looks at various stabilized oxygen delivery systems in greater detail.

Chapter Ten:

Stabilized Oxygen: Introducing Vitamin O

"Oxygen is needed in the body. We can be without food and water for a lengthy time. We can be without oxygen only for a few seconds...It is the spark of life."

Dr. Charles H. Farr, M.D., Ph.D.
O2 Therapies

In view of all the scientific evidence available today, it is clear that an excellent oxygen ratio in the blood stream is a prime requirement for good health. Unlike hydrogen peroxide -- which was the forerunner to these newer oxygen-rich liquid supplements -- SO products hold the oxygen molecules in a stable molecular configuration that typically do not break apart when subjected to heat or sunlight.

Generally, the oxygen atoms are chemically bonded to chlorine salts, like sodium chloride (common table salt -- NaCl). This combination of atoms usually forms a chlorine dioxide compound which is also called " sodium chlorite" (NaClO2).

In order for the body to access the O2 molecule, the sodium chlorite molecule is broken apart by stomach acid releasing the oxygen so that it may be absorbed into the blood stream through the stomach and intestinal linings. This decomposition of the chlorite molecule is quite rapid and the absorption relatively effective.

The current literature explains that nutritional supplements made of stabilized oxygen can be either dissolved molecules of oxygen, (in various molecular configurations including O1, O2, O3, O4, etc.,) or bio-available oxygen molecules electrically bound to numerous salts. These oxygen salts include magnesium, potassium and sodium provided their molecular bonds are easily weakened so that the oxygen molecules may be absorbed by the body into the blood stream.

The literature further explains that stabilized oxygen may be in either liquid or dry forms provided that in the dry form the oxygen molecules may be easily and readily made available to the body.

Many oxygen supplements use oxychlorine or hypo-chloride compounds to stabilize the oxygen molecules. These compounds include chlorite (ClO_2) and chlorate (ClO_3). There is evidence to indicate that chlorite and chlorate may indeed release oxygen in its nascent form as O_2 into the body as these ions are broken down during the digestive process by hydrochloric acid (HCl) in the stomach.

The first report of a stabilized oxygen supplement has been attributed to a solution developed by Dr. William F. Koch, M.D., Ph.D. Reports indicate that one version was used at some point by N.A.S.A. for the space research program, though this report has not been confirmed. Whether true or not, these chlorine dioxide-based liquid solutions would have been ideal for use in space to destroy bacteria and viruses because of the low toxicity of the solution to the astronauts. (42)

Hydrogen peroxide (H2O2) has also been called a stabilized oxygen supplement. Food grade hydrogen peroxide has been used in various formulations for hundreds of years. While it is true that the oxygen atoms of hydrogen peroxide have been "bound" to the hydrogen atoms to form a quasi-stabilized molecule, hydrogen peroxide is not as stable in its electrochemical binding as are traditional oxy-halogen nutritional compounds like the chlorite products on the market today. Hydrogen peroxide easily decomposes when subjected to heat and ultraviolet rays (sunlight). (Again, please see Appendix IX on the use of hydrogen peroxide as an oxygen therapy.)

Dr. John Muntz, D.O., Ph.D., a noted nutritional research scientist, summarized the value of stabilized oxygen in a recent article in *Health World*. He wrote:

"Combine a poor diet with a lack of proper aerobic exercise (low oxygen intake), stress, alcohol and cigarettes, and there are compelling reasons to believe that many of us may be oxygen deficient.

"Can we then improve matters? The answer is obviously -- yes. We can improve our diet, take proper exercise, give up the things that are clearly harmful. But to change our lifestyles or avoid stress may not be so easy

93

to achieve. It is in this context perhaps, that the case for oxygen supplementation is strongest.

"Stabilized oxygen...has been described as the vital nutrient -- vitamin 'O'. But can you simple take it as a daily oxygen supplement? Once again, the answer is yes...What then is the downside? There is none. *(To date, research has not demonstrated significant health hazards from the use of oxygen supplements.)*

"The major constituents and by products have been tested extensively throughout the world without any detrimental effects on humans at the recommended levels. Controversy does exist -- but it is not about the value of oxygen or the safety of stabilized oxygen. The controversy surrounds the micro-biochemical mechanisms that operate at the cellular level, i.e. do the results stem from improved cellular efficiency, through detoxification, better intra-cellular energy transfer systems, enhanced cellular metabolic efficiency, or some of these, or all of these?

"Whatever the answer, if the downside is zero the potential upside is so great that the case for 'vitamin O' as a supplement for our oxygen needs is a very strong one indeed." (48)

Stabilized oxygen supplements are packed with nutrient oxygen that has been called by some scientists and writers as vitamin "O". This oxygen certainly fits the definition of a vitamin, which is a substance found in foods, (or the environment) and is necessary for life, but not necessarily manufactured by the body. Vitamin "O", the oxygen nutrient, Dr. Levine calls the "very spark of life!" (39)

As we've seen, our bodies may be experiencing oxygen starvation on a daily basis. For years, alternative health care professionals have developed and provided natural oxygen therapies to promote healing and well-being. Oxygen alternative approaches to health have been used effectively by these professionals, as reported in over 5,000 published articles, for over 100 years! The research indicates that the following physiological factors rob oxygen from our bodies:

Toxic Stress....Whether derived from the water we drink, the air we breathe or the food we eat, we are now subject to over 70,000 different toxic contaminants, many that did not exist a decade ago. Oxygen is required for the body to even attempt to metabolize and eliminate these lethal chemicals from the body.

Emotional Stress...Adrenaline and adrenaline-related hormones are created by the body during emotionally stressful times (like every day for many of us). The body must use its available oxygen to metabolize these chemicals back out of the body to reestablish metabolic balance.

Physical Trauma & Infections...Bacteria and viruses can put tremendous stress on the body's immune system. When this occurs, the immune system is robbed of the oxygen that is necessary for the body's normal metabolic functions.

Reduction In Available Atmospheric Oxygen...Studies reveal that increased environmental pollution and "green plant" destruction have affected the concentration of the amount of oxygen in our atmosphere over the last 200 years. Many scientists believe that the oxygen content has dropped by over 50% from what it was when the dinosaurs roamed the earth. Others contend that since the advent of the industrial revolution, the oxygen content has declined by as much as three to five percent or more!

Improper Diets...Saturated fats can reduce oxygen in the blood stream. Foods with high fat contents and low nutrient values, like junk and highly-processed foods, have less than half of the oxygen content than do foods containing complex carbohydrates.

Lack of Exercise...Exercising increases the body's metabolic rate as well as the intake of oxygen to help cleanse the body of built-up toxins. A sedentary lifestyle reduces the body's ability to process toxic contaminants and to perform normal functions while decreasing available body oxygen.

Over the last 25 years, extensive lab research studies have been conducted to determine the safety and efficacy of stabilized oxygen supplements. Here is a brief summary of what some of the experts in various disciplines, including the field of oxygen supplementation, have either said or written in the journals:

Dr. James Berg, (paraphrased from "Technical Discussion: Stabilized Oxygen",) states that stabilized oxygen may be found either in its molecular form, primarily O2, and or in an oxygen compound , primarily chlorine dioxide or chlorite (ClO2). (7)

Commonly used oxidants, as described by Brian Goulet, Certified Herbologist in the newsletter (*ALIVE: Focus on Nutrition*: Published by the Canadian Journal of Health and Nutrition), include oxides of oxygen (ClO2, ClO, ClO3, ClO4, etc.), ozone (O3) and hydrogen peroxide (H2O2). (23)

Best-selling author, international speaker and one of the major early authors on oxygen therapies today, Ed McCabe, wrote:

"The so-called stabilized oxygen products are actually salts of oxygen diluted in water. These safe as directed, yet potent oxidizers, sometimes contain various proprietary additives to enhance their effectiveness. They are essentially a formulation mixing a solution of mildly buffered sodium chlorite with deionized water.

"These products are usually weakly buffered to an alkaline pH of around 12% but unlike highly buffered drain cleaners or other strong alkaline solutions, they immediately lose their alkalinity upon contact with any substance that is of lower pH. Bacteria, viruses, the acid mantle of human skin, and the hydrochloric acid in our stomachs all react with stabilized oxygen to immediately render the alkalinity harmless to humans." (42)

Contributing Editor Zane Baranowski in the October 1988 issue of *Health Freedom News* wrote: Stabilized oxygen

"...products are made primarily of chlorine, sodium and water, with extra oxygen stabilized in the the water. This is done by replacing chlorine and/or sodium ions with oxygen molecules. This allows the water to carry larger amounts of oxygen in its whole, stabilized, O2 state. The amount of chlorine in these solutions is small and easily excreted." (4)

James Lembreck, D.C.H., C.M.P. wrote in *Natural Physique*:

"Stabilized oxygen is often confused with hydrogen peroxide, but has a very different action and is very safe to use." (33)

Several years ago, a new generation of stabilized oxygen supplements was released and which has given consumers an even safer approach to increasing oxygen availability in the body. This new formula, was based on dissolved yet completely stable monoatomic oxygen molecules in water rather than oxygen molecules bound to various mineral salts (like sodium chlorite/chlorine dioxide.)

This was a revolutionary concept. The scientific community defended the position that it was virtually impossible to dissolve and maintain more than about 20 parts per million -- ppm (also referred to as 20 milligrams per liter -- mg/L,) of diatomic oxygen in water under ideal laboratory conditions. Yet, test after test, the oxygen levels of this new "breed" of stabilized oxyged indicated levels of dissolved oxygen in the thousands.

This new oxygen stabilizing process was originally developed by a N.A.S.A. engineer and is considered "breakthrough" high technology electrolysis (decomposition) of water into its constituent molecular elements. Regardless of the fact that science says this "can't be done", it appears as though it has indeed been accomplished.

This solution, and its subsequent successor formulations, is also the first stabilized oxygen supplement to claim a nearly balanced pH. pH values express the acidity or alkalinity of a solution on a scale of 1 to 14. Distilled water is considered the neutral "middle point" solution at a pH of 7.0. The lower the pH value, the more acidic the solution is; the higher the pH value, the more alkaline the solution is.

This new paradigm in stabilized oxygen claimed a pH value of approximately 8.5. This pH range is significant in that almost all other competitive stabilized oxygen solutions on the market today, based on the chlorine dioxide (chlorite) molecular oxygen delivery system, have extremely alkaline levels. Hydrogen peroxide-based solutions, on the other hand, have very acidic values. This makes these other solutions potentially harmful when used in full concentration and exposed to the eyes, skin and respiratory system.

Since the introduction of this revolutionary oxygen-rich solution, a family of even more concentrated stabilized oxygen solutions has appeared. Each successor claims it provides even more benefits for specific markets including agricultural, cosmetic, dental, disinfectant and health and nutrition.

Yet, in spite of what appears to be the higher levels of dissolved oxygen in these new solutions, these solutions continue to demonstrate low to non-existent toxicity and high efficacy. Most are sold as proprietary, low sodium, trace mineral and essential mineral dietary supplement formulations.

In a recent limited human-use study on one such solution, conducted by quantum physicist, James Aker, he found:

> "It is the researcher's opinion that *stabilized oxygen* results in greater metabolic efficiency which may correlate to significant energy reductions thus prolonging and enhancing the quality of an individual's life. Further, *stabi-*

lized oxygen, used in conjunction with mineral supplements, may be an excellent therapeutic tool for treating physiological disorders including chronic fatigue syndrome, immune deficiency disorders and several chronic pain related disorders." *

Regardless of the oxygen delivery system, most of the oxygen supplements on the market today, regardless of the technology, offer varying degrees of physiological benefits. Since the release of the first commercial stabilized oxygen supplement called Halox almost 25 years ago, dozens of other products have been introduced for sale to the health and nutrition industry. Many appear to be variations of the same products and merely marketed under different trade names. Others claim to utilize unique oxygen delivery systems containing minerals in various forms.

The three basic categories of stabilized oxygen solutions are hydrogen peroxide, oxy-halogen formulations (including chlorine dioxide/chlorite and magnesium peroxide), and mono-atomic dissolved oxygen. All stabilized oxygen dietary supplements fall into one of these three categories.

*James D. Aker, M.S., P.A., P.P.A., President and C.E.O. of Third State Industries, Inc. Study: "Capillary Martin Microscope Oxygen Saturation Test conducted using Activated Stabilized Oxygen™ (AO2C™) Solution at 100% Full Concentration", April 10, 1998.

Chapter 11:

Human Physiological Uses of and Applications for Stabilized Oxygen Supplements:

"But in the past decade, a broad resistance to antibiotics has begun to emerge. And because bacteria can transfer genes among themselves, experts only expect the resistance to grow. The potential nightmare is an Andromeda strain, a supermicrobe immune to all antibiotics that could wreak havoc. Enter the post-antibiotic era, when people could die of infections that once were treatable."

Andrea Hamilton
Associated Press Release, 1998

Over the last 25 years, stabilized oxygen supplements, either in the form of hydrogen peroxide, chlorine dioxide (chlorite) or as dissolved oxygen in an aqueous medium, have been used for a variety of applications. They have received widespread praise for their beneficial affects.

Applications for the use of stabilized oxygen supplements described in the next three chapters are based on testimonials, research, analytical testing data from lay people and professionals in their respective fields of medicine including naturopaths, nutrition-ists, veterinarians, scientists, agri-culturalists, microbi-ologists, etc.

As mentioned previously, we purposely do not make nor infer any medical claims about the uses of stabilized oxygen for any medical condition, applica-tion or situation. The information that follows is pro-vided for the sole purpose of reporting the uses of all forms of stabilized oxygen.

The reporting of these uses does not imply that the reported specific applications are backed by medi-cal research nor does the inclusion of these uses in this book endorse the use of stabilized oxygen for medical or other purposes.

Acidic Body Chemistry:

Americans are prolific consumers of soft drinks, cof-fee and tea (with caffeine) and red meats. These foods contain excessive amounts of acids which cause sys-temic (whole body) acidity. When the body's pH be-comes acidic, oxygen is needed to neutralize the acid.

As the oxygen is consumed in this neutralization process, the cells, depleted of oxygen, accumulate lac-tic acid and so the cells become acidic themselves. This reduces the amount of available oxygen needed to neutralize the lactic acid in the cells. The result is unhealthy cell metabolism. The regular and daily use of stabilized oxygen may provide the cells with an abundant supply of oxygen to help neutralize the lac-tic acid and support healthy cell metabolism.

Acute Allergic Reactions:

Acute allergic reactions often require oxygen by mouth. The inhalation of oxygen by mouth is only a short-term solution for an oxygen-deficient lifestyle. Repeated and continued use of a concentrated oxygen mixture by mouth may also damage delicate lung tissues. Only a stabilized oxygen supplement is considered safe and effective to use by consumers for this condition.

Angina and Heart Problems:

Physicians have recommended the use of stabilized oxygen for patients suffering from angina and other heart ailments. Many individuals have reported benefits, including the prevention of heart damage after a heart attack, by adding 2-30 drops of stabilized oxygen in pure apple juice and taking it three times a day for several weeks.

Antibiotics and Drugs:

The frequent use of antibiotics and drugs depletes the body of cellular oxygen. An adequate supply of oxygen is required to metabolize these chemicals out of our bodies. Using a supplement of stabilized oxygen may provide the body with added arterial oxygen to reduce or eliminate a toxic build-up of antibiotics and damaging by-products resulting from the consumption of antibiotics.

Bacterial and Viral Infections and Fever Blisters:

Individuals with viral or bacterial infections (including colds, the flu, etc.) in various locations in the body, have suggested mixing 25 drops of stabilized oxygen in a spoonful of honey, taken orally three times daily until the infection clears up. Some individuals with fever blisters (cold sores) have reported that they have applied several drops of stabilized oxygen directly on the sores two to three times a day until these sores have disappeared.

Sores in the mouth have had stabilized oxygen directly applied to the problem areas, on a cotton swab, two to three times a day until the sores reportedly went away. Individuals suffering from Candidiasis have added 10-15 drops of stabilized oxygen to a small amount of natural aloe vera which is applied to the infection until the condition reportedly cleared up. Even some individuals with Herpes simplex on the lips or mouth have noted relief and dramatic reductions in the outbreak, frequency and the severity of this ailment by reportedly using stabilized oxygen directly on the sores.

Reference 1: Sias Laboratories tested the efficacy of stabilized oxygen on three different bacteria: Serratia marcescens, Staphylococcus epideridia, and Pseudomonas aeuginosa. The findings indicate that stabilized oxygen is effective in controlling the growth of these three bacteria. (William Curby, Biophysics Research Unit, Sias Laboratories, Lahey Clinic Medical Center.)

Reference 2: Tests were conducted to determine the disinfectant efficacy of stabilized oxygen on *Staphyloccus aureus, Salmonella choleraesuis* and *Pseudomonas aeruginosa.* It was found that stabilized oxygen demonstrated variable killing power and effective neutralization on the tested organisms. (Nelson Laboratories, Inc., Salt Lake City, UT)

Reference 3: This laboratory analysis tested stabilized oxygen's efficacy on two types of Herpes simplex virus. The findings state the stabilized oxygen does appear capable of inactivating Herpes viruses when the exposure occurs for ten minutes at room temperature. (Department of Microbiology and Immunology, Texas College of Osteopathic Medicine, Louis B. Allen, Director, Virus Laboratories.)

Reference 4: Dr. People's research concluded that stabilized oxygen acts "...as a bactericide and/or fungicide. It works primarily on the basis of oxidation, apparently being able to supply stimulus to the organism's own physiological response as well as offering additional oxidative capacity at the cellular level...Where utilized in vivo, it combines with the natural bodily functions and immune responses to become an effective medication with virtually no toxic sideeffects." (S. Anderson Peoples, M.D., Professor of Pharmacology, University of California, Davis.)

Burns, Abrasions and Cuts:

Both burns and simple cuts can cause trauma to the dermal layer of the skin. This irritation (pain) can be minimized and in some cases eliminated by the application of stabilized oxygen to the burn or injury.

A solution of stabilized oxygen may be applied directly from the bottle or the solution may be added to an atomizer spray bottle for a more gentle and soothing application.

For sunburns or grease burns, stabilized oxygen has been applied immediately on the burn at full-strength. Repeat applications over 30 minutes or more until relief is received and swelling has diminished. Minor cuts and abrasions nay be washed with warm, soapy water and rinsed to remove dirt and debris. Liberal amounts of stabilized oxygen may be applied at full-strength to the wound. Re-applications are made each time wound is dressed.

Superficial cuts may be treated one time with a few drops of stabilized oxygen directly on the cut to help stop bleeding and to reduce the risk of infection. Tests done at Stanford University clearly indicated that stabilized oxygen makes an excellent topical agent. The researchers wrote:

"When applied topically, the product may act as an osmotic agent. The ensuring osmotic gradient would be a sufficient driving force for the removal of toxins from burns and allergenic substances from the skin. In either topical or internal use, this product can act as a non-specific biocide...(it is an) extremely effective viricide, bactericide and fungicide against pathogenic bacteria, enteric viruses, and other viruses." (7)

Reference 1: Stabilized oxygen was tested on 150 patients at General Hospital under the direction of the above doctors to determine its ability to reduce infection and enhance the healing process. The doctors observed that there was an instant decrease in pain among second and third degree burn victims. The healing was especially fast, without infection and without the skin shrinking. The skin appeared smooth and almost looked like normal tissue.

In every case plastic surgery was not needed. They also found that stabilized oxygen prevented infection or eliminated infections especially post-operative where incisions healed in less time than normal. There was an obvious absence of leucocytosis and infection in the area of incisions, leaving a very thin line, without swelling. (Dr. Alarcon & Dr. Garcia, General Hospital, Mexico City. Mexico.)

Cancer:

While tests are certainly not conclusive, there appears to be great benefits for regularly taking stabilized oxygen three to four times a day. Researchers know that cancer cells cannot grow in an aerobic (oxygen-rich) environment. Cancer cells are healthy cells that have stopped functioning as aerobic cells and become anaerobic. (See Appendix VI.)

Large supplies of free oxygen in the bloodstream enter the cancer cells and disrupt the cells' reproductive process and eventually kill the cells. While more research in this area needs to be done, data is available to indicate that a daily consumption of stabilized oxygen may inhibit the growth of cancer cells and promote the growth of healthy blood and body (tissue) cells.

Reference 1: "Dr. Parris Kidd stated that 'Oxygen plays a pivotal role in the proper functioning of the immune system; i.e. resistance to disease, bacteria and viruses.' Dr. Stephen Levine has also stated that 'We can look at oxygen deficiency as the single greatest cause of disease.' thus the development of a shortage of oxygen in the blood could very well be the starting point for the loss of the immune system and the beginning of feared health problems such as cancer, leukemia, AIDS, candida, seizures, and nerve deterioration." B. Goulet, "The Magic of Aerobic Oxygen", Focus on Nutrition. (23)

Reference 2: "Cancer cells originate from normal body cells in two phases. The first phase is the irreversible injuring of respiration. Just as there are many remote causes of plague-heat, insects, rats-but only one common cause, the plague bacillus, there are a great many remote causes of cancer (tar, x-rays, arsenic, pressure, urethane) but there is only one common cause into which all other causes of cancer merge, the irreversible injuring of respiration.

The irreversible injuring of respiration is followed, as the second phase of cancer formation, by a long struggle for existence by the injured cells to maintain their structure, in which a part of the cells perish from lack of energy, while another part succeed in replacing the irretrievably lost respiration by fermentation energy. Because of the morphological inferiority of fermentation energy, the highly differentiated body cells are converted by this into undifferentiated cells that grow wildly-the cancer cells." (Dr. Otto Warburg, Nobel Prize Winner: "On the Origin of Cancer Cells" Science.) (62, 63)

Chronic Sinus Infections:

Some individuals have stated that just 15 drops of stabilized oxygen three times a day in pure water may, by the third day, begin to break up the infection commonly associated with sinus infections.

Douche:

While vaginal tissues are sensitive and delicate, there are reports that a properly diluted concentration of stabilized oxygen in distilled water may relieve many minor irritations including those caused by a yeast infection. The best stabilized oxygen products to use are pH balanced. Reports indicate that for best results, one quarter ounce of stabilized oxygen has been mixed with eight ounces of water in a douche bag. The solution was retained for at least five minutes and then allowed to drain.

Enemas:

Never use any stabilized oxygen product in its full concentration for an enema. The colon and rectal tissues are very sensitive and reports of full concentration applications have indicated that this can cause irritation. The high amount of bacteria in the lower bowels will react to the oxidation potential of the oxygen. Reports indicate that no more than one quarter ounce of stabilized oxygen should be mixed with eight ounces of water in an enema bag.

Environmental Oxygen Starvation:

Scientists have determined that the oxygen concentration in our atmosphere is being reduced at an alarming rate. Some estimates are 0.8% every 15 years. In the 200 years America has been a nation, it has been reported that we have lost almost 11% of the available atmospheric oxygen.

We are "starving" for oxygen in our industrial cities as we breathe the exhaust fumes of automobiles and factories which lock up additional oxygen. We are also destroying life-giving, oxygen-providing vegetation at a rate that is so alarming it is virtually impossible to comprehend. Taking stabilized oxygen supplements may minimize the short-term and long-term effects of oxygen starvation in our atmosphere.

Reference 1: "The body that is oxygen-starved down to the cellular level is in danger of falling victim to disease and injury. Injury is an athlete's worst nightmare; not only can oxygen deprivation contribute to injury, it can also increase recuperation time. Increasing oxygen uptake and utilization by eating a diet high in complex carbohydrates, vitamins and minerals will increase athletic capacity, prevent injury, and decrease the body's tendency toward over-training. The body's ability to metabolize carbohydrates, vitamins and minerals is facilitated by oxygen, enzymes and hormones." (J. Lembeck, D.C.H., C.M.P.., "Stabilized Oxygen...Breathe Easy: Natural Physique.) (33)

Fatigue, Emphysema and Asthma:

Fatigue, emphysema and asthma are conditions where adequate amounts of oxygen cannot reach the bloodstream because of congested airway passages in the lungs. It has been reported that just 15 drops of stabilized oxygen, three times a day in pure water may, by the third day, begin to break up the bronchial congestion and infection always associated with these conditions. Continued and regular use thereafter may begin providing the body with an abundant supply of the vital oxygen for proper cell metabolism. Some asthmatic sufferers, with various conditions, including breathing attacks, have used up to 25 drops of stabilized oxygen in an ounce of pure apple juice for relief.

Reference 1: "Oxygen helps provide us with the energy we need, and the clarity of mind to perform our tasks. It is very important to remember that if we give the body good clean fuel and remain relaxed, allowing it to take in all the oxygen it needs, and barring structural and physiological defect, we can expect good returns in our health and fitness level." (J. Lembeck, D.C.H., C.M.P., "Stabilized Oxxygen...Breathe Easy" Natural Physique.) (33)

Mild Food Poisoning, Diarrhea and Dysentery:

We know that poorly refrigerated or stored foods and unclean water promote the growth of organisms that can cause food poisoning, diarrhea and dysentery. Tests indicate that just five to ten drops of stabilized oxygen in a glass of water has been reported to kill anaerobic bacteria in a matter of minutes. Stabilized oxygen should be taken as an indispensable travel companion. Water contamination is a problem all over the world, not just in the United States. The precautionary addition of stabilized oxygen in a glass of water or juice may prevent a major occurrence of diarrhea and dysentery on that long anticipated vacation.

Food Preservation:

Bacteria grow in an anaerobic (without oxygen) environment. In the refrigeration or preservation of food, the growth of bacteria that can cause food poisoning, diarrhea and dysentery is a possible result. Many suggest mixing 10-12 drops of stabilized oxygen in a half-gallon of refrigerated milk, and that this will keep it fresh for three to four weeks. Others have reported blending 10-15 drops of stabilized oxygen per quart of oil (like olive, safflower, etc.) to prevent rancidity.

Most oils turn rancid not because of the presence of oxygen but because microorganism cultures begin to thrive when they find themselves in an oil-rich nutrient medium. The oxygen in stabilized oxygen retards the growth of anaerobic microorganisms which would normally grow rapidly in such a situation. Oxygen also keeps oils more liquid. When you bubble hydrogen through oil it becomes solid (like margarine or Crisco®). When you submit these same solids to a high concentration of oxygen, they become liquefied again.

Some have blended 14-20 drops of stabilized oxygen for each cup of homemade nut-butters (like peanut or cashew) to prevent rancidity. To keep juices fresh, it has been suggested to add 10-15 drops per quart of juice to extend the freshness several weeks or more.

Insect and Spider Bites:

Just a drop or two of stabilized oxygen directly on a bee or wasp sting,, mosquito, flea, spider or fire ant bite has been reported to bring immediate relief from itching, redness and from swelling.

Increased Stamina and Energy for Athletes and Performers:

Glycogen is the body's chief carbohydrate storage compound. It is largely stored in the liver and, to a lesser extent, the muscles. When we exercise, there is an immediate depletion of glycogen from the muscles. Glucose is the fuel, sparked by oxygen, that is derived from glycogen.

There is a false notion that when anticipating a strenuous exercise we should eat foods high in glucose (sugars) for energy. Rather than high-glucose foods, we should eat high carbohydrate foods. These foods can be easily broken down by digestion to free up oxygen for the body. It is a fact that the most fundamental limiting factor for athletes is cellular access to oxygen.

The American Journal of Clinical Nutrition reported a study that clearly indicated that 48 hours after exercising, a complex carbohydrate diet resulted in significantly higher muscle glycogen levels. Another study in Acta Physiologica Scandanavia demonstrated that the capacity to perform heavy exercises increases 300 to 400 percent when the preceding diet is changed from a low to a high complex carbohydrate diet.

We now know that the cellular metabolism of dense foods like fats and proteins requires extra oxygen from the bloodstream. On such diets, less oxygen will be available for active muscle tissue. Regularly using stabilized oxygen may put an abundant supply of oxygen into the bloodstream for both metabolism and strenuous exercising, and many athletes have reported increased stamina and endurance.

Reference 1: Oxygen is an energy facilitator, enhancer or enabler. In this case the process is called oxygenation; it is the process which energizes the cells for biological regeneration. Without adequate supplies of oxygen, this process-which is at the very foundation of the body's metabolic action-is threatened. Put more simply, without oxygen there can be no nourishment. (Biox Research Limited, Auckland, NZ.)

Kidney, Bladder and Bowel Infections:

Research has shown that kidney, bladder and bowel infections are caused by anaerobic bacteria that grow uninhibited because of an oxygen deficiency in the bloodstream. A dosage of 10-15 drops of stabilized oxygen taken orally three times a day has been reported to be helpful in inhibiting the growth of this bacteria and helping the body's metabolism get back to normal.

Kitchen Uses:

Stabilized oxygen is believed to be an excellent cleansing and purifying wash for fruits, vegetables and meats. Add four to six ounces of stabilized oxygen per quart or water. Dipping fruits and vegetables in this solution has, according to reports, increased their life span for days. Put in a pump spray bottle, this solution may significantly reduce bacteria on poultry, fish and meats when sprayed on them. It is reported that spraying these foods before cooking will reduce the odor and improve the taste.

Plaque Buildup, Gum Disease and Bad Breath:

Plaque is the acid waste matter of bacterial colonies that live in your mouth. As these bacteria eat the small particles of food that lodge between the teeth, they excrete an acid substance which forms the chalky plaque that coats our teeth. Bad breath is also the result of decaying food in the mouth as well as a sign of putrefaction of foods in our digestive system.

To eliminate plaque build up, some individuals report putting several drops of stabilized oxygen directly onto a toothbrush before adding toothpaste. Brush as normal. In between brushings, try gargling ten drops of stabilized oxygen in one ounce of pure (distilled) water to kill the bacteria in the mouth that may cause bad breath.

To eliminate chronic bad breath, some individuals have reported taking 10-15 drops of stabilized oxygen in four ounces of water or juice. This has been reported to kill the putrefying bacteria in the mouth and at the same time puts a substantial amount of oxygen in the blood to kill the anaerobic bacteria causing the problem. (Make sure not to use citric juices like lemon or orange, as the citric acid breaks down the oxygen concentration in the liquid.)

Some dentists have reported using a 30% stabilized oxygen and 70% saline solution injected into infected gums in place of surgery. Others also have reported using stabilized oxygen full strength after drilling and before fillings are put in, to prevent infections.

Polluted Water and Water Treatment:

Our city municipal management and regulatory agencies are reluctant to inform us that our water supplies are dangerously polluted with toxic chemicals, bacteria and other pathogenic organisms including parasites. In fact, research indicates that less than 1% of the water on the planet is pollution/contamination free!

We are told that the levels of these contaminants are below the minimum standards set by the federal government. However, the minimum standards may still be toxic and potentially lethal to human beings if the maximum amount of these minimum levels consumed over an extended period of time.

Studies and news report have revealed instances where much higher concentrations of contaminants have "slipped" through the system and have polluted our drinking water supplies on a regular basis. By the time these "accidents" are caught, the damage has already been done.

Tests have shown that just ten drops of a stabilized oxygen product, in a gallon of water may control coliform bacteria and kill high concentrations of Giardia lamblia in just under two-and-a-half minutes! For campers, hikers, or those storing water for emergencies, just twenty drops of stabilized oxygen per gallon of water has been reported to safely prevent the growth of all bacteria (especially coliform disease bacteria).

Approximately 15-20 drops of stabilized oxygen per gallon of water have been reported to inhibit the growth of disease bacteria. Note that even distilled water, without the addition of stabilized oxygen, may harbor the growth and development of infectious microorganisms.

For water being stored six months to a year or more, some individuals have added one to one and a half ounces of stabilized oxygen per gallon of water. In addition, some have stated that 15-20 drops of stabilized oxygen in an eight ounce glass of water will remove all traces of chlorine and fluorine from water because of the oxidation process.

Note: disease organisms in water can cause severe symptoms and even death. Because there is no simple and quick way to determine the degree and severity of contamination, every precaution should be used in drinking water suspected of containing microorganisms. Whenever possible, drink bottled purified water and add stabilized oxygen as a precautionary measure. Do not be misled into believing that stabilized oxygen alone will kill millions of pathogenic organisms in contaminated water.

Reference 1: "Testing of the antibacterial value of stabilized oxygen as a means of treating water to make it potable and safe is complete. The scientific work has been done by Dr. John Ubelaker, Professor of Biology at Southern Methodist University, monitored by myself. Dr. Ubelaker has now completed the test protocol on bacteria, protozoa, dictostelium fungus, muscle parasites, waterborne cercarie of schistosoma mansoni, and embryonic cells in culture media, and has obtained positive results. With the present data, it is clear that stabilized oxygen efficiently kills pathogenic organisms of interest in rendering water potable." (Baylor Research Foundation, Dallas, TX, J.L. Matthews, Ph.D., Executive Director.)

Reference 2: Professional Services Industries tested stabilized oxygen against a viable culture of Giardia lamblia as evidenced in Laboratory Report #83-533222-1 dated January 10, 1985. Stabilized oxygen effectively kills in just 2.5 minutes 100% of Giardia lamblia concentrations of $1X10(5)$, $1X10(6)$ and $1X10(7)$ organisms/ml of tap water containing just ten drops of stabilized oxygen. At a concentration of only five drops of stabilized oxygen, it took only

3.0 minutes for the culture to be 100% destroyed. (Professional Service Industries, Inc., Arlington, TX.)

Reference 3: On May 4, 1984, Science Research Centre tested stabilized oxygen on five intestinal pathogens. These were: Salmonella typhl, Viberia cholerae, Campylobacter fetus ss jejuni, E. coli (H100407), and Staphylococcus aureus. All of these five pathogens are common waterborne ones which cause the majority of the acute gastrointestinal illnesses that are responsible for the deaths of a large number of children in countries where untreated water is used.

When pure distilled water is innoculated with these organisms, the water requires three times the recommended number of drops (one drop per one ounce of water) to sterilize within three hours. (The high organic content of raw water appears to interfere with the bacterial action of the active components.)

Reference 4: One study indicated that stabilized oxygen treatments can be used effectively to treat contaminated water, though the amount of stabilized oxygen needed to effectively destroy all pathogens is dependent on the amount of organic matter found in the water as well as the total amount of the bacteria present. (Science Research Centre, Abilene, TX.)

Reference 5: "Stabilized oxygen appears to be very toxic to the bacteria, protozoa, fungus and parasitic organisms that were examined. These include:

BACTERIA-Enterobacter cloacae, E. coli, Klebsiella pneumoniae, Salmonella typhimurium, Staphylococcus aureus, Staphylococcus epidarmidis, Streptococcus pyogenes,

Streptococcus faecalis, Proteus vulgaris and *Pseudomonas aeruginosa;*

PROTOZOAN PARASITES-Chilomonas sp., Pandorina sp., Paramecium sp., Chlamdomonas sp., Bleplharisma sp., Giardia lamblia ATCC #30957, Euglena sp., and Euplotes sp.;

PARASITIC ORGANISMS-Nematode parasites of rodents and humans, Trichinella spiralis and *Trichinella pseudospiralis;*

CERCARIAE-Schistosoma mansoni and *Biomphaalaria alabrata;*

EMBRYONIC CELL-Chinese Hamster ovary cells and cancer cells (Hela cells)" (Southern Methodist University, Dallas TX, John E. Ubelaker, Ph. D., Professor of Biology.)

Pools, Hot Tubs and Spas:

Stabilized oxygen may be a natural and safe alternative to chlorine in pools, hot tubs and spas. Stabilized oxygen will reduce algae build-up, keep the pool sparkling clear, and will eliminate the eye irritation of chlorine. Also, chlorine is absorbed through the skin and has been found to be carcinogenic.

The average pool will require a minimum of 55 gallons of pH balanced stabilized oxygen to begin with and then an additional four to six gallons per week to maintain an approximate 30 ppm (mg/L) active oxygen concentration. Stabilized oxygen does not easily break down in sunlight nor by heat as does chlorine compounds, and so has a longer-lasting and safer biocidal/cleansing affect.

Poor Indoor Air Circulation:

Home and office (work) environments become oxygen depleted relatively easily. This is caused by the constant and sometimes excessive use of recirculating air conditioners or heating units. In addition, pollutants (like cigarette smoke), insufficient ventilation and over-insulation may add to this deficiency. The regular use of a stabilized oxygen supplements may give the body the oxygen it needs to function properly under these adverse conditions.

Pre-, Post-Natal and General Infant Care:

Nothing is more important and better for the development of a growing embryo than an adequate supply of oxygen. Research has shown that an excellent oxygen supply to the growing baby during pregnancy will aid in the development of a healthy brain. Stabilized oxygen, in various forms, has been used successfully for over 20 years as a supplement for pregnant women.

A regular and daily dosage of seven to fifteen drops of stabilized oxygen in pure water may provide an abundant supply of oxygen for both mother and growing baby. After birth, one or two drops of stabilized oxygen directly in the baby's milk may benefit a child's metabolism and aid the baby's immune system in fighting off pathogens.

To make sure that the liquids being fed to a baby (under two years old) are free from harmful bacteria, many add one to five drops of stabilized oxygen directly into the milk or juices the baby drinks. For children from three to seven years old, five to ten drops of stabilized oxygen have been added.

Psoriasis and Other Skin Disorders:

Doctors currently treat dermatology problems with a number of therapies including coal tar baths, tar shampoos and other tar topicals, acupuncture, injections and ultraviolet treatments. Many times these prescriptions fail in stopping the spread and in reducing the pain and itch of skin disorders like psoriasis.

Topically applied stabilized oxygen, in a full-strength solution or just a few drops in cold water, has had remarkable results. Patients have seen dramatic and rapid improvements including the reduction in the size of the inflammation, the severity of the itching discomfort and a loss of pain.

Also, 20-50 ounces of stabilized oxygen in a bathtub of very warm water is reported to bring relief for a variety of skin problems including rashes, eczema, psoriasis and athlete's foot. The problem areas should be fully immersed in the water for a minimum of 20 minutes and this process should be repeated three to four times over a period of a week.

Reference 1: Dr. James D. Berg, Ph.D., of Stanford University's Department of Medical Microbiology, determined some potential mechanisms for stabilized oxygen as a therapeutic agent. "First, when applied topically, the product may act as an osmotic agent. The ensuing osmotic gradient would be a sufficient force for the removal of tox-

ins (i.e. from burns, allergenic substances, etc.) from the skin. Second, in either topical or internal use, this product can act as a non-specific biocide.

"Both stabilized oxygen and one of its reaction products, chlorine dioxide, are extremely effective virucides, bacteriacides and fungicides against pathogenic bacteria (e.g. Legionella pnuemonphilia), enteria viruses (Poliovirus) and other viruses. Third, potential mechanisms of this product involves utilization of chlorite by the cells, particularly leukocytes, as a substrate to increase the efficiency of the a group of enzymes known as peroxidases, which are an important component in the immune system since they are involved in the oxidation of foreign material (e.g. viruses).

"This product significantly improves the efficiency of the two enzymes chloroperoxidase and peroxidase. These three possible mechanisms are, of course, not exclusive of one another. It is quite probable that all three act simultaneously." (Stanford University School of Medicine, Stanford, CA, Department of Medical Microbiology.)

Reference 2: In tests done at the University of Illinois, it was determined that stabilized oxygen contains a substrate that will support enzymatic halogenation. The research indicates that the substrate is chlorite. Dr. Hager concluded: "If there is a similar enzyme or enzymes on the surface of the skin or in the bacteria or fungi themselves, you have a good basis for the antimicrobial activities...That mechanism would be the generation of an enzyme-bound chlorinating species which would be very toxic for microorganisms. In humans, in the white blood cells, there is an enzyme called myeloperoxidase which kills ingested microorganisms by a similar chlorination process." (Dr. L. Hager,

University of Illinois at Urbana-Champagne, School of Chemical Sciences.)

Stress:

Any stress, whether caused by infections, toxic chemicals, emotions, or physical trauma, results in the dramatic increase of free radicals in the cells. These free radicals steal the available oxygen. Free radicals are highly reactive molecules considered by many researchers to be the primary cause of aging.

Stress, especially if it is prolonged, depletes the cells' oxygen supply. This predisposes the individual to a host of diseases and illnesses including cancer. The continued and regular use of a stabilized oxygen supplement may aid cell recovery during times of stress.

Toxic Chemicals:

Unfortunately, our environment is polluted by toxic chemicals (like pesticides, herbicides, hydrocarbons, and solvents.) These chemicals, (they are fat-soluble,) eventually find themselves in the food chain in nutritious foods that should provide us with the pure and untainted vital nutrients for a healthy body. Yet, as we digest these potentially toxic foods, the toxic substances enter our bloodstream and wind up in our cells.

To free our bodies of these toxic chemicals, our bodies utilize oxygen to metabolize these toxic substances. But this metabolic process depletes our bodies of much of the available oxygen at the cellular levels. The regular and daily use of a stabilized oxygen supplement may provide our bodies with additional oxygen to replace the oxygen consumed in this cleansing process as well as providing us with an abundant supply of oxygen for healthy cellular metabolism.

Vaporizers:

Those suffering from respiratory problems note some relief when adding four to six ounces of stabilized oxygen in one gallon of water in a cool mist vaporizer. A wide variety of conditions such as emphysema, chronic obstructive pulmonary disease, bronchitis, and pneumonia have responded well to this type of application.

Yeast Infections:

Bodies with poor oxygen supplies available to the cells have been found to be more susceptible to common yeast infections such as Candida albicans. Because of the low oxygen environment in many individuals, Candida albicans thrives.

Candida is an anaerobic (without oxygen) loving organism. One of Candida albicans' waste products is a substance that is responsible for cellular damage (acetaldehyde).

Acetaldehyde in the intestinal wall and liver will disrupt the intestinal absorption process of nutrients. The red blood cells do not get needed minerals, vitamins and other nutrients, and the lymphocytes cannot function properly to attack invading pathogens like Candida. The regular and daily usage of stabilized oxygen may give the body the needed oxygen to repair damaged cells and to energize the immune system.

Reference 1: This research project tested the efficacy of stabilized oxygen on inhibiting the growth of Candida albicans and Saccharomyces. The findings indicate that stabilized oxygen does retard the growth of both yeast species. (Daniel Tuse, President, Toxicometrics Incorporated, Sacramento, CA.)

Chapter 12:

Agricultural and Horticultural Uses of and Applications for Stabilized Oxygen Supplements

"As we consider the environmental effects of various hurtful and hazardous chemically caused problems, we ask, 'Is this an inevitable situation? Does progress necessarily include negative effects? If our land and our health suffer from the results of our activities, is restoration and healing possible? If so, how? What will be required, and what must we do?'"

Dr. William R. Jackson, Ph.D.
National Award-Winning Author
Environmental Care & Share

As mentioned previously, oxygen comprises almost 50% of the soil and 50% of all vegetation on the planet. It is a critical ingredient in all plant metabolism since oxygen interacts with the minerals and beneficial microorganisms in the soil as well as the root systems of every living plant.

Agricultural animals (horses, cows, pigs, chickens, etc.,) whether as a food source or used for recreational or other uses, require the energy produced from the consumption of vegetation. These grasses and grains contain high amounts of oxygen, an element that is required for plant respiration. This supplemental source of oxygen, taken internally, also provides the same basic physiological benefits to animals as it does to humans.

The carbon dioxide and oxygen cycle of plants is a remarkable biochemical phenomenon and yet, at the same time, a delicate system of balances. Plants take water from the soil and carbon dioxide from the air and convert these molecules to simple sugars in a process called photosynthesis.

Without the green pigment "chlorophyll", plants would not be able to absorb solar energy from sunlight to complete this process. One of the waste products of the photosynthesis process is oxygen.

Dr. William Jackson, Ph.D., a noted author, educator and researcher on both hyperbaric oxygen, oxygen and plant nutrition and organic soil conditioning wrote:

"With each molecule of carbon dioxide assimilated to produce organic compounds, the plant gives up a molecule of oxygen which was donated from the splitting of water molecules. It has been hypothesized that all the oxygen in the atmosphere originated in this manner. Scientists have determined that if photosynthesis were to stop abruptly, all free oxygen would become nonexistent in a few short years because the carbon cycle would have been disrupted." (29)

Stabilized oxygen can and does provide beneficial oxygen for agricultural and horticultural uses. These uses include dips, washes and food supplements for livestock and agricultural crops. Stabilized oxygen is also an excellent soil enhancing agent.

Algae and anaerobic microbial build-up in drip irrigation systems is a function of the low oxygen content of water through the system which gives rise to anaerobic conditions that are favorable to organisms that contaminate and damage irrigation systems. Stabilized oxygen may used as an oxygen enhancer to the flow of water through these systems to increase oxygen levels in order to retard the growth of such organisms.

In addition to its anti-microbial properties, stabilized oxygen may also provide oxygen-rich water to the plant root systems enhancing the aerobic plant growth (respiratory) cycle. Plant tissues require free oxygen for life -- just like the oxygen in stabilized oxygen solutions containing bio-available diatomic oxygen. Aerobic respiration plays a critical role in providing metabolic energy to all higher plants. Oxygen, plus sunlight, results in tremendous amounts of metabolic energy as the end product of photosynthesis.

Reports also indicate that combining stabilized oxygen in irrigation water along with low molecular weight fulvic acids may significantly increase the uptake of oxygen. In fact, research indicates that concentrations of 50 mgl $^{-1}$ of fulvic acid in a nutrient solution causes the uptake of oxygen in the root systems of tomato plants to increase over 38%! Similar results were observed in sugar beets.

Generally, the amount of oxygen that can be maintained in water depends on water temperature, salinity, atmospheric pressure and microbial concentrations. Colder water holds more oxygen. As salinity increases, oxygen retention decreases, that is, fresh water contains more oxygen than does sea water. Both the partial atmospheric pressure and the degree of oxygen saturation of oxygen in water will change with altitude since gas solubility decreases as the altitude increases.

Microbial content plays a key role in the loss of oxygen from water, especially surface waters. Microbes use oxygen as energy to break down long-chained organic molecules into simpler and more stable end products such as carbon dioxide, water, phosphates and nitrates. As organic molecules are broken down, oxygen is depleted from the system. The higher the content of organic matter in water, the greater the microbial growth and the greater the degree of oxygen depletion. Finally, flowing water contains higher levels of dissolved oxygen than does standing or stagnant water.

Dissolved oxygen levels are one of the most important parameters in aquatic systems. Oxygen is absolutely required for aerobic organism metabolism and oxygen also influences inorganic chemical reactions. Adequate levels of dissolved oxygen are needed and are necessary for excellent water quality. As dissolved water levels drop below 5.0 mg/L (5.0

parts per million/ppm), all aquatic life is subjected to stress. The lower the oxygen concentration, the greater the stress. Oxygen levels that remain below 1.0 to 2.0 mg/L for a few hours can result in the death of large numbers of aquatic life. The ideal range of dissolved oxygen in water should be in excess of 5.0 mg/L and not fall below this level.

Current research indicates that minimum dissolved oxygen levels in water should be at the following concentrations:

Warm Water Fish: 5.0 ppm
Cold Water Fish: 6.0 ppm
   Spawining Fish: 7.0 ppm
Estuarine Biota: 5.0 ppm
Recreational Lakes and Streams: 3.0 ppm
Drip Irrigation: 5.0 ppm
Bioler Feed Water: 0.1 to 1.4 ppm

The control of micro-organisms and algae in water corresponds to the existing oxygen saturation levels in water and the level of contamination in the water supply. Thus, the higher the contamination of the source water and the lower the existing dissolved oxygen concentration, the more stabilized must be added to bring the delivered water to the appropriate minimum usage ranges.

Antiseptic Dip:

Approximately 1 ounce of stabilized oxygen in one gallon of water can make an effective antimicrobial dip for fruits and vegetables. Stabilized oxygen acts as a topical disinfectant for surface disease organisms. Tests indicate a high destructive organism ratio - on contact - against most anaerobic molds, yeasts, fungi and bacteria.

Flowers, Foliage Plants and Ornamentals:

Flowers, foliage plants and ornamentals are susceptible to a variety of diseases like powdery mildew, black spot and rust. A 50% stabilized oxygen and 50% water solution, in a spray bottle can reduce and in most cases eliminate these problems. Reports of stabilized oxygen used on roses suffering from these blights indicate a complete elimination of these problems in only two applications. The upper and lower surfaces of the foliage were sprayed in the early mornings or late evenings for best results. This spray is also effective on powdery mildew on snapdragons, beans, peas and strawberries.

Foliar Feed:

Add one gallon of stabilized oxygen to 30 gallons of water as a foliar feed. This mixture is sufficient to spray one acre of plants. Spray on plants early in the morning (4:00 to 8:00 a.m.) when the plant pores are open. Excellent results have been reported when used on soybeans, edible beans, corn, wheat and oats.

Frost Resistance:

Current plant research indicates that when oxygen-rich water is added to a foliar feed spray on potatoes, this new solution enhances the plants' resistance to frost damage down to as low as minus 5 degrees Celsius. Treating potatoes at five and one quarter quarts of stabilized oxygen in 20-30 gallons of water per acre, plus the foliar feed (three pounds of dry soluble powdered foliar feed), resulted in a yield of six tons of potatoes per acre, mainly due to the fact that the treated potatoes continued to grow in spite of the frost, and that the untreated potatoes were frosted-off at the soil level.

General Agricultural Applications:

Diatomic oxygen and ozone are also found in rain and snow which supply vital oxygen to all plant life. Research indicates that the oxidation process appears to stimulate protein production in growing plants. The benefits of higher oxygen concentrations in water supplies to vegetation include thicker plant stems, larger leaves and shorter stem internodes.

In standing crops, such as potatoes and corn, plant stems are thicker and stronger and the leaves are a brighter green color than those not receiving additional oxygen. Oxygen-nourished plants are believed to be more drought and disease resistant (especially to root-borne pathogens).

House Plants and Cut Flowers:

All house plants can benefit from an increase in oxygenation. About seven teaspoons of stabilized oxygen added to two gallons of water will enhance the opening of flowers. Using 15 drops of stabilized oxygen in a vase of fresh cut flowers will keep the water fresher and clearer, will enhance flower appearance and life (up to 50% longer!), and will encourage flower opening. (Please note: soft tissue plants, such as tomatoes, should not be misted or sprayed with this mixture, as direct applications may result in scorch marks.)

Orchard Use and Fruit Set:

Spraying fruit trees at petal fall with full-strength stabilized oxygen may enhance fruit set. Subsequent sprays promote a higher growth rate, and the flavor of the treated fruit, when compared to untreated fruit from the same orchard, shows improvement in both quality and flavor.

Some reports indicate that watering the ground around fruit trees with a 50% solution of stabilized oxygen may increase fruit yield. In some cases, trees that had not produced fruit for several seasons bore fruit once again.

Seed Germination:

To help germinate seeds, add eight ounce of stabilized oxygen per 16 ounces of distilled water. Soak the seeds for eight hours before planting. Some experiments with old wheat seeds resulted in an astonishing 90% germination rate compared to a control soaking in water that yielded only a 60% rate of germination. Non-productive rice paddies have also been reactivated by the addition of stabilized oxygen using the same formula.

Drinking Water for Farm and Ranch Animals:

One gallon of stabilized oxygen in 1,000 gallons of water will increase the dissolved oxygen level in the water to approximately 35 ppm (mg/L). This mixture ratio may be used for all farm animals including cattle, swine, poultry, sheep, goats, and rabbits. When used in this ratio for dairy cattle, results indicate an increase in milk production and butterfat content with reported less mastitis (an inflammation/infection of the udder) in the herds.

Hog farmers report a shorter time preparing hogs for market, with an increased weight gain with less feed used. The drinking water is reported to be cleaner and fresher, with a noticeable reduction in algae, bacteria and rust. There appears to be some control of the outbreak and spread of animal diseases.

Dairy Uses:

The use of stabilized oxygen in dairy farming was first recorded in 1985. At that time, stabilized oxygen was added to the polluted water system of this one particular farm whose situation was further complicated by an outbreak of mastitis in the herd.

The farmer recorded a significant reduction in the occurrence of mastitis as well as healthier cows. By 1988, the butterfat content of his cows had increased by 5.3%. Other farmers have reported production increases as high as eight pounds of butterfat per cow per milking, with bacteria counts as low as 2,000 per cubic centimeter.

Stabilized oxygen can be used in the same way as a pipeline rinse for milk stone, depending on the length of the pipeline. As a rule, 14-24 ounces of stabilized oxygen should be added to 15 gallons of water, and used as a rinse. This ratio may also be used to rinse milk cans and the bulk milk tank to reduce bacteria levels.

Stabilized oxygen may also be used as a completely safe and non-toxic udder wash in a ratio of eight ounces of stabilized oxygen to one gallon of warm water. Cows have soft, tender teats, and a dissolved oxygen-based formula of stabilized oxygen will not irritate the teat ends. The solution may be placed in a pump spray bottle and sprayed directly on the teats and the udder as often as needed to help reduce bacterial infection.

Stabilized oxygen can be used as an additive to colostrum milk to reduce spoilage until it is to be used to feed newborn calves. Though the pH and temperature of the milk will vary, it is generally recommended that two ounces of stabilized oxygen be added per one gallon of colostrum milk.

Newborn calves need extra oxygen. To facilitate this, add two ounces of stabilized oxygen to a bottle of calf milk twice a day (morning and evening). This appears to "brighten up" the calves, and in some cases reduces scours (diarrhea due to dysentery), which can lead to dehydration and/or death.

Reports also indicate that stabilized oxygen, when added to the water of cows that have just calved, appears to "clean out", (i.e. help to discharge out all of the placenta and afterbirth,) these cows much faster, thereby avoiding the infection resulting from a retained afterbirth material.

An oxygen-rich drench can be used for cows with high fevers or for off-feed cows with mastitis. A solution of 14 ounces of stabilized oxygen to one quart of water should be used as a drench in the morning and in the evening over a three day period.

In addition, stabilized oxygen may be applied directly to wounds on the skin surface to enhance the healing process.

Crop Residue Converted to Animal Feed:

Stabilized oxygen can be used to convert crop residue into cattle feed. Residual crop items (straw, corn stalks, corn cobs, soybean residue, etc.) may be treated with a direct application of stabilized oxygen. Mix one part of stabilized oxygen to 34 parts water and soak the residue material for 16 hours.

This soaking process appears to breakdown the fiber materials so that these materials may be more easily assimilated. Some feedlots have reported that the meat quality on animals fed using this process to be as good as those animals fed a diet of only corn.

Slurry Tanks:

Slurry tanks are used by farmers to store animal

wastes, usually wastes from dairy barns or hog operations. Odor is often a problem with these storage tanks. Research indicates that adding approximately 120 gallons of stabilized oxygen to every 350,000 gallons of slurry, and then agitating the slurry, will significantly reduce slurry odor. In some cases, the odor may even be completely eliminated.

Fertilizer Use:

For field use, a truck tanker car of black strap molasses and digesting bacteria should be added to slurry tanks four days prior to applying the treated slurry to fields as a fertilizer. In addition, 120 gallons of stabilized oxygen should be added two days prior to application and dispersion on fields, and the entire solution should be agitated before application. The resulting solution has been reported to be odor-free and is an exceptionally fine fertilizer.

One gallon of stabilized oxygen may be added to one gallon of black strap molasses in 20 gallons of water per acre to use as a spray fertilizer enhancement to winter wheat crops for a higher and faster yield.

Another farmer injected a solution of one gallon per acre of stabilized oxygen with 10 gallons of water with his corn seed at planting time. Even during a drought year, he harvested 130 bushels per acre, indicating that this mixture may have provided a measure of drought and stress protection to his crops..

There is some research that indicates that treating herbicide-contaminated soils with a 50% solution of stabilized oxygen and water, over a two week period, may help neutralize these toxins. It is believed that the oxygen in this solution oxidizes the toxins and allows sensitive plants to grow in soil where previously they could not grow.

Chapter 13:

Animal and Pet Care Uses of and Applications for Stabilized Oxygen Supplements:

"What is man without beasts? If all the beasts are gone, man would die from great loneliness of spirit, for whatever happens to beasts also happens to man. All things are connected. Whatever befalls the earth befalls the sons of the earth."

Chief Seattle of the Suquamish

Stabilized oxygen supplements are extremely potent and effective broad spectrum natural bactericide, fungicide, antiviral, and antiparasitic compounds. They are environmentally safe with no toxicity to either man, fish, reptiles or animals.

Aquaculture/Fish Farms:

Stabilized oxygen may be used as a bactericide and fungicide in both pre-harvest and post-harvest treatment. Add 160 drops per gallon weekly for optimum bactericidal effect. Reports indicate that when added to water, the fungal growth rate in the tanks and on the fish is significantly reduced. A solution of approximately five to ten ppm of pH balanced stabilized oxygen will yield noticeable results. Tropical fish breeders have added one to two ounces of stabilized oxygen to 20 gallons of aquarium water to control microbial and algae growth.

Bird/Aviary Cage and Feeder Wash:

Stabilized oxygen is a mold inhibitor, is antibacterial, antifungal, antiviral and antiparasitic. Wash feeder units with 50%-100% solution prior to each feeding. Stabilized oxygen can be used as an effective yet completely safe antimicrobial cage wash. Stabilized oxygen and sodium perborate were used by Robert Stroud (the famous "Bird Man of Alcatraz") to heal birds as reported in his book <u>Diseases of Birds</u>.

Reports have been made stating that 10-20 drops of stabilized oxygen, added to hummingbird feeders, will reduce or eliminate fungal and bacterial growth around feeder tube openings. The addition of an oxygen solution appears to act as a natural preservative, keeping the sugar solution fresher so that it will last longer.

Fresh or Salt Water Treatment:

Stabilized oxygen may be used as a disinfectant for both aquarium and/or contaminated water, as well as an additive to water to inhibit microbial or algae build up. Add 80-160 drops of stabilized oxygen per one gallon of water depending on how much contamination is in the water.

Hogs:

Research indicates that stabilized oxygen added to the drinking water of hogs results in meat that is more lean than the meat from hogs fed untreated drinking water. In some cases, hog fat content has been reported to be lower than 10% of total body weight.

Hogs are susceptible to various diseases, including pneumonia. These diseases are held in check with the use of various antibiotics. Stabilized oxygen appears to reduce the need to use large doses of antibiotics. Also, hogs that drink water treated with stabilized oxygen are reported to have healthier respiratory systems and are subject to fewer diseases.

Hogs with scours (diarrhea due to dysentery) have been treated with a solution of approximately one half ounce of stabilized oxygen per gallon of drinking water for three days. Then the mixture was reduced to approximately 15 ounces of stabilized oxygen per gallon of water for maintenance.

Poultry:

Tests indicate that stabilized oxygen added to poultry drinking water may reduce the outbreak and severity of the avian flu virus. In addition, stabilized oxygen has been reported to increase egg production in those hens drinking water so treated, having a higher oxygen content. Some poultry farmers have reported that chickens drinking treated water have reduced incidences of breast blisters and the heavier chickens have a significant reduction in tendon breakage.

One turkey farm in Canada reported that its birds had a lower mortality rate, consumed 8 1/2% less feed, yet averaged 1 1/2 pounds more weight per bird because of the use of oxygen treated drinking water.

Washing boiler carcasses in stabilized oxygen has been shown to reduce the levels of salmonella contamination. One study, reported in Poultry Science (Issue 66, 1987) resulted in a noticeable reduction in salmonella after a ten minute dip in a 1% solution of stabilized oxygen.

In another test, broiler carcasses were soaked for ten minutes in a 50% solution of stabilized oxygen and water. Tests indicate that the salmonella bacteria levels were reduced and in some cases completely eliminated.

Reptiles:

Stabilized oxygen may be used as an antimicrobial disinfectant wash for reptiles, reptile cages and as a hand wash for pre- and post handling. Use from full strength to 50% strength. A pump spray bottle should be used for best dispersion.

Feeders and Feeder Units:

Stabilized oxygen may also be used as a mold inhibitor, as well as an antibacterial, antifungal, antiviral, and antiparasitic wash for feeder units. Wash feeder units and tanks with a 50%-100% solution prior to each feeding or filling as a natural, yet safe, disinfectant.

Appendix I:

Consumers Praise the Benefits of Stabilized Oxygen Supplements!

Please Note: The author and publisher make no medical claims about the use of stabilized oxygen for medical purposes. The testimonials that follow were, to the best of our knowledge, unsolicited from consumers who have approached their health ailments and needs by using stabilized oxygen as a dietary supplement instead of, or in addition to, traditional medicines, over-the counter remedies or accepted surgical or medical procedures.

As the largest chapter in this book, these testimonials are provided for the sole purpose of sharing what consumers are saying about stabilized oxygen supplementation. Neither the author nor the publisher wish to imply that these testimonies are backed by medical research, nor do we endorse the use of any stabilized oxygen for any medical purposes or problem. Again, this is what consumers from around the world are saying about the benefits of various stabilized oxygen supplements on both individuals and animals.

All references, in the following testimonials, to specific brand name products, manufacturers or distributors have been replaced by the generic name "sta-

bilized oxygen" to prevent the endorsement of any one brand or company over another.

The Testimonials...

"I have been on antibiotics off and on my whole life and I have suffered from Candida. The only way I am able to keep it in control is with *stabilized oxygen*. I now have more energy and less fatigue." *B.S., UT*

"Rusty, our huge and magnificent tabby, came to us, like all our pets, as an orphan in need. He was about two years old and accustomed to fending for himself. We healed a large abscess under his chin by cleansing and spraying the area with a two% solution of *stabilized oxygen*. We treated his snake-bitten paw, swollen to triple size, with the same solution. Both healings were complete within two to three days, as was a deep cut between his eyes." *E.S., AZ*

"I was diagnosed with the Epstein-Barr virus and suffered from tremendous headaches and serious fatigue. After going to a regular M.D., I finally received my first dose of *stabilized oxygen* from a homeopathic specialist. The headaches began to subside and the fatigue gradually improved...The *stabilized oxygen* now gives me more energy and my whole body feels much less fatigued." *S.K., UT*

"I have absolutely no hesitation in recommending *stabilized oxygen* to my patients as an integral part of their overall therapies to rebuild their immune systems and metabolic processes. It has proved to be completely safe and I have had no incidents of complications. I highly recommend *stabilized oxygen* as a daily supplement for everyone, not just those who have health problems." *K.H., D.C., D.I.C.A.K., UT*

"I have suffered with poison oak every time I ride out in the mountains. I rubbed a *stabilized oxygen* solution of about one quarter *stabilized oxygen* with three quarters water, and overnight, the poison oak was gone! *D.M., CA*

"Last year my son sent me a bottle of *stabilized oxygen* and I started taking the product immediately. Over a four month period I gradually increased my dosage from seven drops to 55-60 drops a day. I can now work outdoors four to six hours a day without an asthma attack. I seldom, if ever, use my atomizer and I think *stabilized oxygen* has also increased my levels of energy, alertness, and has improved my memory." *T.O., OR*

"Hot grease that splashed on my hand-I used *stabilized oxygen* on it with cotton balls until it quit hurting-approximately 15 minutes. All the pain was gone and there was NO SCAR!" *R.E., UT*

"Last week I was in agony when a patch of psoriasis (covering the entire instep and ankle of my left foot,) became infected, swollen and bleeding. This happened in spite of using every ointment, herbal tea remedy imaginable. I prepared a two percent solution of *stabilized oxygen* and immersed the entire foot for 25 minutes. All night I continued to feel pain. But by morning a great change had taken place! No swelling! No pain! Foot healed overnight! Glory be! *M.P., CA*

"I have a severe chronic inflammatory condition that began in my late twenties. This condition has caused severe headaches, chronic fatigue, digestive problems and at times I am barely able to move, although I am not chronologically old...I have tried many alternative remedies but until taking *stabilized oxygen* had not seen such immediate positive results. I have been taking *stabilized oxygen* for 10 days. Prior to this I was having a severe flare up, but due to complications had been told to avoid medications. Ten days may not seem like a long time for a test, but for me a week without pain is like a miracle. I am not exhausted all the time and have more energy. It has been great being pill free." *M.E., CA*

"My mother suffers from migraine headaches and has been taking *stabilized oxygen* for several months. During this time the headaches have stopped. When she ran out of *stabilized oxygen* for several days, the headaches started up again. Needless to say, she takes *stabilized oxygen* on a regular basis." *J.J., CA*

"For 14 years, I have battled "Athlete's Foot", and, despite the best of the over-the-counter remedies, such as Lotrimin, and the much stronger prescription salves, I was always on the losing side of the battle. Even after following all directions (multiple applications/day for 2-3 weeks), the fungus always came back in the form of red, itchy spaces between my toes, and, much of the time, the red/itchy areas only diminished and never really disappeared. I decided to try *Stabilized Oxygen*. I began with lightly rubbing 5-6 drops into each of the "infected" areas, once in the morning, and again at bedtime. In just 3 days I noticed improvement, and decided to continue the same treatment regimen. Within eight days, I neither saw nor felt the Athlete's foot. No more itchy feet! Now to keep the fungus at bay, I apply the *Stabilized Oxygen* drops only once a day, and I have yet to see in the 9 weeks any more of that irritating problem. WHAT A RELIEF!" *J.R., NV*

'I have eczema on my hands. I have tried other products, but nothing has worked. The *stabilized oxygen* has given me relief. As soon as the eczema starts to flare up, I use the *stabilized oxygen* and the itch and rash never materialize." *P.L., CA*

"Besides *stabilized oxygen* being used as an internal bactericide, viricide, and fungicide, it can be used topically for burns and rashes. Also it can aid in combating parasites...It can be used to improve almost all health problems." *Dr. C.L., Ph.D., N.D., UT*

"Stabilized oxygen has increased my alertness and energy levels. Smoking took my breath away and *stabilized oxygen* gave it back." *E.N., CA*

"I am a marathon runner. My PR is a 3:08:0 at the 1993 St. George Marathon. Prior to that time, my PR was a 3:16:20 (also at the St. George Marathon). I attribute this improvement to the use of *stabilized oxygen.* My training, weight, and all other factors were very similar as I checked my training logs. I have to attribute the eight minute improvement to *stabilized oxygen.* I just felt better!" *J.D.B., UT*

"Last week, while cleaning my garage, I picked up an empty milk carton and felt a sudden sting on my hand. When I turned the carton upside-down, a small black spider tumbled out, and I stepped on it promptly. I assume it was a black widow spider, very common in this area. I hurried into the house and applied *stabilized oxygen* concentrate directly on the bite area. Within five minutes the pain was gone and the red streak up my arm was no longer visible.." *V.R., AZ*

"With regular *stabilized oxygen* use and increased dosage immediately before a race, I have noticed increased endurance, strength and aerobic capacity. I look forward to my first long course competition in the San Luis Wildflower Triathlon next May." *L.S., CA* (nationally ranked triathlete)

"I suffer with a rather rare variety of lung disease which has severely impaired my right lung. *Stabilized oxygen* seems to help so far." *W.B., SD*

"Late in the day last Tuesday (July 22) I noticed that my son Adam, five years old, had a few bumps on his face and chest. We had been sitting on the lawn so I assumed they were bug bites. The next morning he woke up with a raging case of chicken pox. He looked as though he had been boiled; bright red from his chin down to his feet, his feet so swollen that he could hardly walk, oozing pustules on his thighs, arms, chest and buttocks, dark red welts where ever his skin creased. He was tormented with itching and cried off and on for hours, complaining that he was on fire. At mid-morning I put him in a tepid bath, tub fairly full, with about two cups of *stabilized oxygen* added. This helped somewhat....When I spoke with the nurse at the doctor's office I was told that chicken pox runs about seven days. The next morning, Thursday, Adam bounced into our room at the crack of dawn singing and dancing...and feeling his usual self. All of the redness was gone and the only indication that he had had chicken pox were the dried and healing pustules. By Friday, these too were gone." *S.S., OR*

"My sinuses, which have been infected since about 1940, are under control. They still discharge pus, especially now in the hay fever season, but it no longer makes me ill. My asthma, which dates back to the same period, is almost totally gone." *Rev. P.D., CA*

153

"I can't thank you enough for introducing me to *stabilized oxygen*. This miraculous product has definitely improved my sense of well-being. I feel more energized, less nervous and feel confident that *stabilized oxygen* has reduced the harmful toxins in my body. I have applied it directly to my skin to relieve the pain caused by burns and bites, and I feel that I have lost weight as a result in taking your product. I can never thank you enough." *G.T., CA*

"I can tell you that *stabilized oxygen* has eliminated a painful plantar wart from the ball of my left foot thereby obviating laser surgery. I am delighted! *B.R., CA*

"I wish to express my gratitude for your product. It seems my heart wasn't getting enough oxygen and after consulting my doctor I gave *stabilized oxygen* a try. It, plus the herb hawthorne, saved me from taking digitalis for the rest of my life. I am 75 years old and feel young again. I wish everybody could have some of this wonderful *stabilized oxygen*! *V.J., CA*

"During the past year, I have had several bladder infections, sometimes reoccurring after two weeks. Previously, I had gone to the doctor and received a prescription for one of the sulphur-based drugs... On one occasion during the summer, when I realized another infection was coming on, I took ten drops of *stabilized oxygen* in an eight ounce glass of water before going to bed, rather than taking the prescription drug. In spite of the discomfort, I was able to go to sleep and I awoke the next morning without a trace of the bladder problem." *M.M., NY*

"My son Jon brought me a couple of bottles of *stabilized oxygen* when he came home for Christmas. The last four years I have been in the hospital 34 times, not counting the times I just went to the E.R. I've had angiaplasty 12 times and I didn't have the energy to even do my housework. The last time I was in the hospital was just before Christmas. When I take *stabilized oxygen* for my angina, I feel better very quickly. I was on oxygen for a long time. Because of *stabilized oxygen*, now I don't have to carry an oxygen tank with me and I can go places I've not been able to go to in a long time. Best of all, I haven't had any chest pain for three months! I'm sending you a picture taken a few months ago. I will be 76 years old Friday and I feel like a spring chicken thanks to *stabilized oxygen*. Even the age spots on my hands and arms are clear now that I have been putting *stabilized oxygen* on them." *H.R., AZ*

"My husband had an ugly mole on the back of his leg for 10 years. It was about 1/2 inch across. Lately, it had begun to turn strange colors and puff out about 1/8 inch, so now it was catching on his pants when he put them on and removed them. This caused tearing and bleeding. We were getting quite concerned about the negative change in this mole. We tried everything we could think of, but nothing worked. We even tried the Colloidal Silver, but there was no improvement. Then we tried the new stabilized oxygen. The results were definitely worth sharing. We put the *stabilized oxygen* on a cotton ball and secured it over the mole with a Band-Aid. We resaturated the cotton about 3 times a day -- morning, after work, and bedtime. The first week, absolutely nothing happened. The second week, it started to turn even more colors and to dry up. The third week, it just fell off! After all these years -- end of mole, end of story. I'm sharing this because I would like to help others who might be considering freezing, cutting, or burning off such a nuisance and potential cancer problems. Try stabilized oxygen first. You might also be pleasantly surprised!" *L.S., WA*

"My husband has suffered with asthma so severe that it was classified as "life-threatening -- the most dreaded category in which to land. He was totally steroid dependent in order to control it. We lived in an area of North Carolina that was full of industrial pollution, and the problem was further aggravated by massive amounts of pollens of all kinds drifting in from the Blue Ridge Parkway.

"We also learned that we can put it directly into the nostrils and use it like nose drops, or fill a nasal spray bottle and spray up the nose. It relieves congestion and the often resulting sinus infection that can cause an overabundance of mucous. He always used to carry a nasal spray bottle to help him keep breathing, but no longer. Another thing we learned as we shared our experience, is that we can fill a spray bottle and spray the *stabilized oxygen* toward the back of the throat and inhale. His Prednizone is now down to 3 mg per day, and considering that he was at 100 mg., you can imagine how grateful we are!" *D. C., WA*

"For 3 years I couldn't have any air blowing on me. I wore a heavy coat summer and winter. I couldn't use my air conditioner. It gets 95 here for four months in the summer. I was given a bottle of your *stabilized oxygen.* In one week's time I was better. In 2 week's I was completely healed. Also my arthritis is much better. I tried every vitamin that they sell. Nothing helped. I took 20 drops morning and noon. I am 84 years old. I can't thank you enough for your *stabilized oxygen.*" *R.P., TX*

"I am a retired accountant, and for a long time I have suffered with severe pain in my elbows, forearms and shoulders. About four months ago I started taking *stabilized oxygen.* I started at 20 drops 2 times a day, and had no results. Then I increased it to 30 drops 3 times a day, in water. I experienced dramatic relief, and so I kept it at this level for 6 weeks. Then I decided to see if I could get the same results without using so much, so I dropped it to 20 drops 3 times a day, and still had the same results. So now I take 20 drops per day and am still doing just fine. I guess I just had to use a bit more to get enough in my system after years of being oxygen deprived.

"I have also dramatically reduced my medications for asthma by using the stabilized oxygen...I no longer need Prednizone. The year before I discovered your products I was in the hospital five times, and I have had no bouts that would land me there since being blessed with these formulas. Being a senior citizen, you can't imagine how grateful I am that you have helped me save my breath, my health, and my money!" Thank you. *L.T., WI*

"From earliest childhood, I have had every form of bronchial problems. After using *stabilized oxygen*, I am off antibiotics and inhalers. I am feeling much better with additional energy. I would recommend *stabilized oxygen* to anyone with any form of bronchial problems." *J.G., LA*

"In July I started taking 20 drops of *stabilized oxygen* three times a day. Here are the results so far: After 4 days the cramps in my legs and feet stopped. Also the soles of my feet stopped burning. After 6 days my eyes were clear of burning and itching...After 5 days my stomach cramps disappeared. After 7 days -- I've had manic depression for 30 years. With lithium, sometimes I have a few flashes of fantasy. It is gone. After 7 days -- I've had emphysema for 13 years. My breathing has improved, both day and night and I have no pain. After 7 days -- my stool has become normal. The best in 10 years -- frequency, substance, and ease. After 16 days the occasional problems I've had with my prostate have disappeared...After 21 days, no pain or joint restriction to any bone. After 3 weeks I feel like a new man." *M.S., TX*

"A year and a half ago my doctors prescribed thyroid medication. Soon after I started taking this medicine, I developed a bad cough. I believe I may be allergic to the medicine, but three different doctors I consulted told me to keep on taking it. So for the past year and a half I have been coughing everyday. I'm so happy I found *stabilized oxygen!* In less than a week my coughing stopped. I took 10 drops three times a day to start. Now I only have to take 10 drops a day and no more coughing! Thank You." *E.R., FL*

"I was born with food allergies and so it came as no surprise when I got asthma after eating a small pat of butter that kept me out of school for three weeks. So I began with health problems and they multiplied. Chronic fatigue ... Headaches ... Sinus, were some of the things I suffered from, but the worst part was a feeling of terrible fatigue. My fatigue was worse after eating. It felt like someone hit me in the pit of the stomach and knocked all my air out. Then I would have to lie down for a while until I recovered. After getting my first bottle of *stabilized oxygen* I took 21 drops and waited to see what would happen. WOW!! I could breathe through my nose! I thought it was just to hold my glasses. What a difference! I have ENERGY.

"Before everything was very hard to do, so much so that even after taking a shower, I had to lie down to catch my breath. Now I feel human again. I now walk two miles to the grocery store each day. It used to take me an hour - now just 40 minutes. I still have plenty of energy so sometimes we go to the mall shopping till 9 PM when they close. I'm walking 105 steps a minute and feel GREAT! I'm 68 on the way to 100." *K.E.H., UT*

"Cuts on my hands or face usually show redness and infection and take a long time to heal. *Stabilized oxygen.* clears them in hours and they heal in a couple of days. Gargling with a few drops stops gum infection and pain. I love it! Took a skin cancer off my nose. It just dried up and I scraped it off!" *M.F.*

"I took 10 drops of *stabilized oxygen* twice the first day it came and I woke up the next morning pain free for the first time in a few years. I am going to keep on taking it, as it is such a relief to be pain free. Now I can shop and do things my painful back and hips never let me do before. I actually spent a whole day Christmas shopping this year. And I was able to do things the next day." *E.B.*

"I took a 3-1/2 hour flight from Detroit to Phoenix in December. When I arrived in Phoenix, a severe headache hit me as I walked up the ramp. I believe that this was due to the lack of oxygen and fresh air during the flight and therefore my body needed oxygen! I carried a bottle of *stabilized oxygen* with me and put about 50 drops under my tongue and after 30 seconds washed it down with some water. Within 3 minutes the headache went away as fast as it came on. I gave my body what it needed." *J.E.*

"My sister received a newsletter on stabilized oxygen. We were both trying to find something to help our Dad who was battling numerous health difficulties and on an inhaler and bedridden most of the time. I started Dad on *stabilized oxygen*, 30 drops twice a day. He is no longer on the inhaler. By the second dose of stabilized oxygen I had more energy. After four days the intense pain left my thighs, hips and arms and has not returned. I believe my body was full of toxic poison from undigested food that got in my blood. L. G., MO"

"I use stabilized oxygen twice a day and it keeps me off the breathing machine. If I miss using it for a day or two then I realize how much it helps. Then I start wheezing and am more short breathed and can't do as much." *W.B.*

"After taking *stabilized oxygen* for several months (20 to 30 drops per day), I find I have more energy and stamina, have become immune to colds and flu and the people in the office plus my family comment on how good I look and they are surprised to discover I'm almost 69. That's wonderful for the ego! " *J. C., TX*

"In March of 1997 I had a diagnosis of cancer in both lungs. I was told that surgery was the only solution because neither chemotherapy nor radiation were an acceptable option, because of my poor condition. I had some emphysema and a plugged main artery in my heart, and they weren't sure I'd make it through surgery. If I did nothing, I wouldn't live any more than six months to a year. I told them if I was going to die, I was going to die whole. In August I went fishing in Canada with my two sons and my youngest grandson. While sitting and talking one evening all of a sudden I pitched forward and was not breathing and had no heart beat. My youngest son gave me CPR while the oldest went to call an ambulance. Our grandson Casey PRAYED. In the hospital they found I had very low potassium, down to 2.5. For 30 hours they gave me potassium intravenously. After leaving the hospital I was very weak and staggering all over. I used a cane for about a month.

"One day while seeing my chiropractor, he told me he had just read an article and the first person he though of was me. I asked him what it was. He said *stabilized oxygen*. I asked at several health food stores and none had heard of it. Finally my chiropractor got some in and I was there when it came. Three days after starting the *stabilized oxygen* I threw my cane away. In November we went to Arizona to our park and I bought myself a bicycle. No one had expected to see me back...Now every day someone comes to my door because of how I look and act, wanting some of this *stabilized oxygen*. I take 30 drops 3 or 4 times a day and no medications. I take other vitamins and minerals, but I never leave home without *stabilized oxygen*. In December the x-rays showed that both tumors were getting smaller. This is a long way from the doctor telling me to get into the Hospice program in August." *H.C.L.*

"In January of 1968, when I was 41 years old, I suffered a massive embolism of the lungs. After weeks in the hospital I went home, but I have never been able to do much of anything since then. After 10 minutes or so I have always had to stop and rest. I never could hurry or run or walk upstairs without stopping and resting. Now with taking a few drops of *stabilized oxygen* about 3 times a day, I am a different person. Thank you so much!" *M.G.*

"My husband George, who is 96 years old, has clogged arteries in his legs. This has bothered him for several years. He could walk only about 100 feet, then stop, because of the severe pain in the muscles in his calves and thighs. After a few minutes rest he could walk another 100 feet or so. Our doctor said this was happening because the muscles were not getting the oxygen they needed due to the clogged blood vessels. We tried many supplements, but nothing happened. When I read about *stabilized oxygen* in a newsletter, I sent for it. I gave my husband 18 drops in 7 ounces of bottled spring water, twice a day, before breakfast and a half-hour before dinner. It took three months to be effective. Now he can walk a half-mile, sit for 10 minutes to rest and then walk back home without pain. My husband also has severe arthritis in the lower spine due to a bad fall on icy pavement four years ago. He no longer complains of the pain and he stands and walks straighter since taking stabilized oxygen. P.S. We have been married 72 years. (I am 87 years old.)" *A.I., NJ*

"I have been taking *stabilized oxygen* for six months. It has improved my life 98%. I have had chronic bronchitis since 1962 (36 years!). I coughed most of the time. Since being on the *stabilized oxygen*, I no longer cough. It's a miracle! I am 68 years young. I thank the Lord every day for *stabilized oxygen*." D.S., Florida

"I used *stabilized oxygen* on my husband's diabetic ulcers (sores) on his foot and within two and a half weeks they were all healed up, whereas no doctor could get them to heal. As for myself, I use 15 to 30 drops in water each day. I noticed I can go up and down stairs much better than before. Also a hump I had on my neck below my back skull is gone. Now I can turn my head better. Also my neighbor thinks there is nothing better for cuts and scratches." *R.H., UT*

"For several years, my 10-year-old granddaughter had a warty area in the web between two fingers, which interfered with daily use of her hand. Various home treatments included drugstore remedies, trimming, hydrogen peroxide, aloe gel, aromatherapy oils and minerals solutions, but nothing was completely successful. It eventually became the size of a nickel. Her pediatrician said it was "the worst kind of wart" and used Histofreeze on it. Still, it returned. Then dermatologists cut it out and used liquid nitrogen - all of this involving pain and extensive recovery time. Still the wart returned! She then I began to rub *stabilized oxygen* on it twice a day, and the skin became normal in one month. She is careful to keep an eye on the area, and still uses the *stabilized oxygen* several times a week for prevention. Personally, I rub *stabilized oxygen* on those horrid age spots, and find that they lighten." *J.R., NH*

"I'm really pleased with the results I've had in using *stabilized oxygen* for "dry eyes!" I'm finally rid of this irritating condition after two and a half years. When I feel it coming on I take 20 drops under the tongue and within minutes it's gone. Great Product!" *J.H, ID*

"I reached my 89th birthday on February 20, 1998. I was born with a "shunt" (a hole) in my heart and am the only person so afflicted to live beyond 50 years. The New England Medical Journal will confirm. I had moderate emphysema (from smoking for 71 years), an enlarged heart, and problems with my bronchial tubes and pulmonary arteries. I have been taking stabilized oxygen...twice a day for 6 months and have experienced sensational assistance. I walk briskly and can sing like a lark!" *S.S., FL*

"Your *stabilized oxygen* is indeed amazing. I have an allergy to smog, and get severe ear infections...My allergy to smog was severe enough to cause a brain hemorrhage 30 years ago, and I had to move more than once, to elude the smog. With *stabilized oxygen,* I can stay where I am and enjoy daily living." *F.B., CA*

"My mother was suddenly diagnosed with severe blockage of the main arteries and doctors would not operate due to the possible consequences of such an operation. Soon my mother was bed-ridden to the point where she could not even get out of her room because she was too fatigued and tired and in need of her oxygen tank. Then I found out about *stabilized oxygen*. I sent a supply to her and in three days she was up on her own, no more oxygen tank, running errands, cooking just like normal." *W.G., CA*

"When I read that *stabilized oxygen* removes seborrhea from the scalp it was almost too good to believe. I have had seborrhea all my adult life. I took 30 drops of *stabilized oxygen* in pure water three times a day between meals. The very first week the awful stuff cleared up. I keep taking it in smaller amounts now." *E.P., OR*

"I work at an astronomical observatory on top of Mauna Kea, here in Hawaii. There is only 60% of the oxygen normally found at sea-level. I had read about *stabilized oxygen*, so a few months ago, I ordered three bottles... and started using it daily. I take about twice the recommended dosage. I notice a definite increase in energy, mental clarity, and ability to perform strenuous tasks at this high altitude. I have not noticed any negative side effects." *J.C., HI*

"After biopsy surgery on September 25, 1997, the miasma and surrounding area were not healing as well as I hoped. After five months, there was a mass under the skin. The incision was dark red and Vitamin E seemed to heal it only so far. There was frequent discomfort and pain. I began to apply *stabilized oxygen* to the area in March. The discomfort decreased after just a couple of applications. The scar resumed healing. Two months later, the mass has greatly diminished in size...the scar is smaller. I can also testify to the effects of ingesting the *stabilized oxygen*. On the treadmill, I could only walk about 7 minutes, with *stabilized oxygen*, I walk 20 minutes!" I.S., AZ

"*Stabilized oxygen* has been wonderful for me. I've been taking 15 drops twice a day for several months now. My thinking has never been clearer and my intuition has sharpened greatly so that I'm seeing things more clearly and making better decisions. I'm also sleeping better and the content of my dreams doesn't drag me down anymore." M.W., CA

"*Stabilized oxygen* makes me feel so good! It reminds me of the Miracle Grow I give my plants, but this *stabilized oxygen* is for me!" D.P., N.M.

"I bought a bottle of *stabilized oxygen* just to see if it would work. I have had headaches for more than fifteen years. It is caused by a benign tumor behind my right ear. No operations of any kind, says the doctor. He has tried all kinds of medicines, no cure. I put 25 drops of stabilized oxygen in a glass, poured some distilled water into the glass and stirred it with a plastic spoon. Bingo, two hours later my headache was gone. I can even see better, and my hearing is a little better too." *W.F., N.C.*

"My father who is 76 years old had gotten a very bad chest cold. He felt so weak he wouldn't have any visitors. I gave him a bottle of *stabilized oxygen* and after a week he was back to his old self. He takes it every day now. My husband has a friend that had emphysema and he got tired just walking up or down stairs. My husband told him about *stabilized oxygen* and the man bought some. He called about three weeks later and said it was working very good for him - so much so that he now walks about seven blocks a day and feels great." *L.B., PA*

"It seems incredible that just 40 little drops of *stabilized oxygen* in a glass of water daily has made me a new woman! I feel completely renewed in body and mind and also uplifted in spirit. At 84 years old, I live life enthusiastically and joyfully, looking forward to each day's tasks as well as rewards. I'm in close touch with, and adore my two grown children and my grandchildren. Frequently I play winning bridge at my club, so obviously this keeps me mentally alert. So, what more could one want!" *M.W., FL*

"I had a burn, 1/2 inch by 1/4 inch, on my hand from touching the hot oven rack. It had been there for approximately two years. It would scab over and then peel, leaving a redness, sometimes to the point of al-

most bleeding. One day when I was taking *stabilized oxygen* internally, I put a drop on this area. After putting a drop on daily for about 5 days the area was noticeably healing. Another 2 days and there was only a very light area of redness; only noticeable to myself."
Dr. S.C., MA

"I cannot in all honesty say enough about what *stabilized oxygen* has done for me. I had a touch of emphysema and had to use two inhalers three times a day and I used to wheeze also. Then I took *stabilized oxygen* to see if it would work and found to my amazement that it did! I felt really good and had a sense of well being that I hadn't had in years. I found I needn't depend on my inhalers anymore and my wheeze went away. I could breathe again like I used to. Thank you for *stabilized oxygen*." *G.C., TX*

"I have been using *stabilized oxygen* for six months now and have lots of energy. It clears up cuts in no time. My husband is 77 and is diabetic. He uses it every day also and has lots of energy. Plus it cleaned up the ulcers on his feet which no doctor could do. It's a wonderful product which we will never be without."
R.H. , UT

"I want to say thank you for letting me know about *stabilized oxygen*. It sure is great and I sure do feel super. It got rid of the gas I've had for a long time. Of course I've been on vitamins for years, but *stabilized oxygen* is the best. I hope I never run out of it. I don't feel as achy in my joints as before. I sure love it. I also give it to my husband. He has a chemical imbalance and by taking it he is much better."" *F.P., MA*

"I tried *stabilized oxygen* to see if it did everything that it was claimed it could do. I have fibromyalgia and one of the most annoying problems is a "fuzzy" brain. *Stabilized oxygen* has given me a much clearer brain function, more energy and has lessened my pain. My husband has COPD and the *stabilized oxygen* has eased his breathing difficulties so he can be more comfortable." *A.G., N.C.*

"I take 20 drops of *stabilized oxygen* each morning. Recently I had a breaking out of running sores on my right hand. Some of the remedies I tried without success were hydrocortisone, Benedryl, comfrey poultices, Vitamin E, sulfur and lard, and potassium permanganate. I started using *stabilized oxygen* every three hours and my hand is now doing very well. The itching and weeping have gone away."*E.R., MI*

"*Stabilized oxygen* has relieved the pain and redness of my right hand. Before starting to use *stabilized oxygen* I was rubbing my hand in pain medicine and wearing gloves at night. I no longer wear the gloves. My breathing is much better and this allergy season has not been rough by using *stabilized oxygen*. I have more energy and am able to do more as my arthritis pains are not felt like before." *H.C., W.V.*

"Thank you for your product *stabilized oxygen*. It has given me back my life. Four years ago I suffered a heart attack brought on by severe asthma. The past four years have been spent searching and trying every product I could find. Some helped, most didn't. I heard of *stabilized oxygen* from a friend. Now after two bottles and one month I am living again! The chest pains are gone. The asthma is now a rare occurrence. I look forward to taking *stabilized oxygen* every day of my life. It has made such a difference. Life is now exciting and wonderful again." *K.D., CA*

"I have been taking *stabilized oxygen* for about three months. I am diabetic and before I started taking *stabilized oxygen* my legs used to hurt very bad when I walked. My legs stopped hurting the day after I started taking stabilized oxygen and have not hurt me since. My wife has introduced our neighbors to it, and they also have had positive results. I live in an elderly housing project and all the people here are either elderly or disabled." *J.H., HI*

"*Stabilized oxygen* - what a fantastic product! After taking it, I now don't need my Claratin and Vancanase A.Q. for my asthma. I had asthma for six years and this is the best I have felt in ten years! *Stabilized oxygen* also heals cuts. Four weeks ago I had a cut, bad enough for stitches. I put some *stabilized oxygen* on it and the cut is now almost gone." *D.M., PA*

"I was disabled last October with lung cancer...I could not walk 50 paces without stopping. My breath and legs would give out. I read about *stabilized oxygen* and decided to get some. I have taken it for about four months. It's a Godsend. My legs don't give out anymore; my breathing is 25% better. My blood pressure also dropped. I feel so much better. I don't even think of my condition. I'm telling everyone about *stabilized oxygen*." *I.W., W.V.*

"I have heart disease. I am undergoing alternative therapy (chelation), in addition to taking various supplements. *Stabilized oxygen* has made a large difference in controlling my angina. I am able to reduce it or even prevent it. I am recommending *stabilized oxygen* to anyone suffering from respiratory or cardiovascular problems. I find I get the fastest relief when taking the *stabilized oxygen* sublingually." *Dr. U.B., MI*

"I want to take a few lines to praise that wonderful *stabilized oxygen* you make available. I had originally purchased it for myself to aid me in this pollen season here in Ohio. When I first received it I was fairly "stuffed up" in my sinuses. After 7 or 8 drops I waited patiently hoping to see some difference, any difference in maybe 5 or 6 hours or even the next day. I was pleasantly shocked to find that in just a few minutes (about 5) my breathing was normal again. I was truly ecstatic. That night I placed the bottle of *stabilized oxygen* by my bed in case I needed some during the night. By around 6 AM my son (who is 5 years old) came to me and said "Mommy, Mommy, I can't breathe!" The *stabilized oxygen* came to my mind and I gave him 5 drops under his tongue. It worked even quicker on him (about 2 minutes). Now when he wakes up and his nose is stuffed he just asks me for the *stabilized oxygen.* I've also given the *stabilized oxygen* to my 80 year old Dad when my parents visited us recently. Since their visit was 2 weeks long, I thought it would be a perfect opportunity to give some "life" back to my Dad. You see, Dad has a history of heart problems and has been very weak and out of breath. Dad noticed a difference in the first day. By day 5 he was riding my Schwinn Airdyne Exercise bike for 5 minutes with its oscillating handle bars." *N.W., OH*

"I have been a diabetic for over 22 years and have always had a problem with my vision. After taking *stabilized oxygen* for just a short time, my vision has improved tremendously. I am very pleased with the results." *L.F.T., AL*

"I have two little four-legged critters, cockapoos. One is nearly 14, and the other is almost eight years old. I apportioned them a dosage of *stabilized oxygen,* based on their weights relative to mine, and I'm glad to say that the older one is much more peppy, her breath is sweeter, and the tongue of each of them is distinctly pinker (as in more oxygen in their circulatory system.) Since I don't know the color of my tongue before I started taking stabilized oxygen, I can make no comparison!! My vet recently saw the older of the dogs and could hardly believe that she was the age that she is. She runs all over the place, jumps up on the sofa, and goes right over the arm at the end, down to the floor, and repeats a loop around the living room. She's like the Energizer Bunny! So, you can be sure that I will continue to take *stabilized oxygen* and give it to my dogs..." *J.S., CA*

"My husband has diabetes and his leg used to hurt him so much when he walked. But since he has been taking *stabilized oxygen*, all of the pain has gone. His sugar count is great. He feels great. Now where he works, they all want to start taking the *stabilized oxygen*. I can only say that this is the best thing he has ever taken to help him." *L.H., HI*

"In 1996 and 1997 I was very short of breath all the time. My oxygen level would get in the low 80's and I felt BLAH! I have had asthma all my life, and was always using inhalers, pills galore, and going to the doctor every month. My diabetes was in bad shape. My sugar count was always in the 300 range, and got as high as 600. I took insulin shots, and medication and the level got down in the 180 to 200 count range. In early 1998 I heard about *stabilized oxygen*. I ordered two bottles.

"After 90 days I had my oxygen level tested, and it was 97%. My oxygen level stays in the mid to high 90% range. Today my blood sugar count is in the 90 to 120 range, depending on my diet. My oxygen stays in the high 90% range, and I take no medication of any kind. I am 70 years old. I wish I had known about *stabilized oxygen* 25 years ago. Now I can enjoy hunting, fishing and gardening without shortness of breath and wheezing like a winded horse.

"I haven't been to the doctor in 5 months. I am a firm believer in *stabilized oxygen*. Presently I am taking 30 drops twice a day in a small amount of water, then drinking a glass of water following the small amount of water with *stabilized oxygen*. I have lost 25 pounds the past year and I'm feeling great! *H.V.*

"I am 70 years old and have tried many products with no perceivable benefits. I only have a small Social Security pension and it is difficult to buy all the nutrients I am told I should be taking. I have been unable to take a deep breath for several years. I have practiced for some time forcing air into my lower lungs 20 times, then forcing it into my upper lungs 20 times, but I could not get it into both parts at the same time, and could not get the air into the very top of my lungs. After taking *stabilized oxygen* for one month, I woke up the next morning and took a deep breath and filled my lungs with air, clear to the top! Now I practice taking deep breaths several times a day." *P.D., OR*

"I have read many of the testimonials of people using stabilized oxygen. Nowhere did I see an example of simply rubbing the stabilized oxygen on painful areas. I tried this with an arthritic joint of mine and the pain stopped instantly!! I couldn't believe it!" *R.C., NY*

"I thought I would share with you the best piece of news in the whole world. I am a 56 year old woman and have been hooked on nasal spray since I was 28. Not just any spray but the strongest 4-way Menthol. None others would work. I used two to three bottles a week. I have been using *stabilized oxygen* for about 3 weeks. Yesterday it occurred to me that I didn't use the 4-way even once and last night I used a saline moisturizing spray one time. Today I didn't use it again. This is a miracle! The E.N.T. I saw a few years ago told me that I would never get off nose spray. Thanks a million. Never stop making stabilized oxygen. It is incredible. It has also been helping my husband's lung problems." *J.S., ID*

"I was developing a cataract in my left eye. I decided that if *stabilized oxygen* is safe to take by mouth it surely could not harm my eye. Imagine my amazement when the second day of using a drop twice daily I could tell a difference. I have now finished my first bottle and my problem is almost totally gone. Thank you for *stabilized oxygen*." *E.P., CA*

"How can I say "Thank You?" You have given back my life! Nearly five years ago, I became very ill and suffered debilitating pain and fatigue. After several months of expensive testing I was diagnosed with lupus, possible co-mingled with scleroderma: two incurable, potentially fatal diseases. I was 24 years old. We began aggressive treatment of my symptoms, and I gained a measure of relief, but was still unable to work a job or give my family 100%. I still suffered from constant pain and bouts of severe fatigue. Then about six weeks ago, my grandmother introduced me to *stabilized oxygen*, and my whole life changed. Here a few of the things that have changed: I sleep soundly without being awakened by pain; I wake up refreshed and energized; my photo-sensitivity has improved dramatically; the dark circles under my eyes are gone; I put in 16-18 hour days and don't spend two weeks in bed recovering; I have energy to do things I thought I would never do again; the constant pain I have lived with the five years has lessened considerably; I am now working full-time plus going to college two nights a week, plus taking care of two young children. I would never do it without *stabilized oxygen*. From the bottom of my heart, I thank you!" *N.C., FL*

"I have been taking *stabilized oxygen* for about two years now. It helps keep Candida under control...By the way I am 83 years old." *V.S., CA*

"I wish I had known about stabilized oxygen years ago. I started taking *stabilized oxygen*...about three months ago. I am 86 years old. I could hardly get out of bed from back pain. I also had lots of pain in my right shoulder. It was so bad I couldn't raise my arm to comb my hair. I am much better now." *Y.H., CA*

"*Stabilized oxygen* - what a product. Everything you need in one little bottle. It has really changed my life. I now have energy to keep up with all the young guys at work. And even beat them at pole top rescue. (I work for the electric company.)" *J.H., CO*

"I am 80 years of age and have terrible lungs and was having asthma attacks day and night for a long time. I received some literature about *stabilized oxygen* about five months ago and I ordered four bottles and have been taking it since that time. Am I a believer? I swear I have not had even one attack since starting on it. I was on Theodurr and Albuterol inhalers. Three inhalers per month. Now I have almost forgotten about Theodurr and inhalers..." *I.D., LA*

"I have had blocked arteries for a long time. I also have emphysema and lung disease. The doctors told me that my left lung was the size of a 12 or 13 year old and my right lung was not working at 100%. The pain in my chest would put me back in the hospital again and again...I have not had any more chest pain at all." *C.B., N.C.*

"*Stabilized oxygen* has worked wonders. After using it for two months I noticed a profound difference in my breathing. I am so grateful that I discovered such a worry-free and simple remedy, helping me with my hay fever." *A.S., FL*

"I had seven surgeries to remove tumors in the bladder. But my May 27, 1998 the doctor said there was nothing more he could do but remove the bladder. I talked with my family doctor and he suggested a second opinion. At my age, 85, I didn't see how I could go through the surgery of removing the bladder. This is when I ordered...*stabilized oxygen.* Three months later the doctor took a scope and found five small tumors, which he removed..." *O.F., OH*

"I work as a telescope system specialist for the James Clerk Maxwell Telescope on Mauna Kea, Hawaii. The high altitude of this facility, almost 14,000 feet, means there is only about 60% of the oxygen at sea level. Your *stabilized oxygen* has boosted my energy level and alleviated many of the negative side effects of working at this high altitude." *T.L., HI*

"Of all the vitamins I have taken, and still do, none has produced the miraculous changes that *stabilized oxygen* has done for me. I have only been taking it for a short time, but already I can tell the difference. I use to be very unsteady when I walked, today it is as if I had taken 20 years off my age. I used to awaken two or three times every night, short of breath, it was frightening. Now I have perfect rest. Truly, I can't say nearly enough in praise of this wonderful stabilized oxygen." *L.P., NV*

"I'm 66 years old and every day after lunch, I would take a little rest. Now after taking *stabilized oxygen* I don't feel I need to take an afternoon nap anymore." *R.R.S., WA*

"In 1997 I found I had Myelo Dysplastic Syndrome. It is a rare condition of faulty red blood cells causing anemia. I have been taking *stabilized oxygen* for one year and I feel better than last year. My eyesight also seems to be getting better. I take 30 drops four times a day and when I feel tired I take 10 drops by mouth. I believe this is keeping me going." *J.M., OH*

"My wife has advanced alzheimers. I have been giving her an average of 30 drops twice a day. There is some indication that is doing some good, so I will continue to order more. I have started to take it myself and feel it is cleansing the colon and giving me more energy." *W.W., OH*

"I am 64 years old and had been a caretaker for many years. It left me drained and without energy. I also encountered some health problems in the last 2 years. I took other vitamins but they did not work well...In the state of health I was in it took about 3-4 weeks to feel a difference. However, since then I will not be without it ever again. Now at least I feel better than I have felt in some time. My general health has improved and I am able to walk better without the constant aches and pains from arthritis." *M.G., NY*

"*Stabilized oxygen* has helped me in several ways. Taking it before bedtime keeps my sinuses open for the night. It is also helping my kidney problem and I am gaining in strength. It is a very valuable vitamin."*V. M., MS*

Appendix II:

Oxygen in Cosmetics and Dental Products

Oxygen, in one form or another, has been used in a variety of consumer products in the cosmetic and dental industry for dozens of years. National brands have advertised that their products contain oxygen. F.D.A. (U.S. Food and Drug Administration) restrictions prevent these manufacturers from really explaining to the public why oxygen has been included. We're left to making assumptions about the benefits or just ignoring the reference to oxygen as just another wild marketing claim without substance.

The truth is, oxygen does have a major role to play in these industries. More and more research is being completed revealing the beneficial, disinfecting and cell enhancing properties of oxygen. With this in mind, let's take a more serious look at oxygen and its role in cosmetic and dental products.

Since Ponce de Leon's famous journey to the Americas, the search for the Fountain of Youth has been the focus of cosmetic manufacturers around the world. The cosmetic research journals contain one study after another claiming that they have finally uncovered a solution that prevents or reverses the skin aging process. Perhaps the most important thing to establish is that we cannot reverse the aging process. It is an inevitable fact of life.

As we age, our body's ability to control free radical production diminishes and it is the inability to control these atoms and molecules that causes the aging process. Any claim of a miracle "cure" is completely misleading.

However, we can minimize the effects of aging on our cells and body. We've already discussed how important oxygen is to the cells and how a lack of oxygen can actually increase free radical production. We've also discussed the importance of taking supplemental antioxidants to help control or "deactivate" free radicals. Therefore, products that contain both antioxidants and oxygen would be of great value in minimizing skin aging.

Dr. Paul Herzog, M.D., one of the great pioneers in studying the skin aging process and its relationship to oxygen deficiency, wrote:

"The main reason for the premature aging process in facial skin is that the subcutaneous cell tissue, which should regularly receive sufficient oxygen and nutrients by fluid exchange between blood plasma and the interstitial fluid, receives inadequate amounts of these nutrients and oxygen even as early as puberty, presumably due to insufficiency. The oxygen deficiency arising in this way can be so important that the facial skin can no longer maintain its young and healthy appearance. The biological processes involved must therefore be given assistance in compensation for the deficit of oxygen and vital nutrients such as vitamin A, glucose and water, so allowing the skin to maintain its young appearance."

There are no blood vessels in the outer layers of the skin. Capillaries are responsible for providing these layers with nutrients and oxygen. However, circulation in these capillaries declines rapidly as we get older. They become less permeable and so less oxygen and nutrients pass from the capillaries to the extracellular fluid which surrounds the cells.

Healthy skin is balanced with oxygen, nutrients, good capillary circulation and excellent lymph drainage. The ability for the skin to repair itself or to maintain a youthful look is directly proportional to its ability to receive nutrients and oxygen from the capillaries.

The body has a remarkable cleansing process called the lymph system which is designed, in part, to remove wastes from the skin cells. If the cells cannot get enough oxygen, the toxic wastes will build up in these cells, and the lymph system will not be able to remove them adequately nor completely. As waste products of metabolism as well as toxins accumulate, the skin cells, once soft, supple and pliable, now become dry, brittle and eventually die.

Dry skin is dehydrated skin. As we age, the dermal layers (epidermis) thins out. As it thins out, water is more easily lost from these cells. As the water evaporates, the dermis becomes dry, wrinkled, lined, blotchy, less elastic and less healthy. It also loses the oxygen that is dissolved in this water, oxygen that is crucial for the normal metabolic processes of these cells. As we have also noted, oxygen is also the perfect cleanser. It kills detrimental microbes (including bacteria) that attack these skin cells, as well as other organisms that try to invade the cells themselves.

Moisturizers -- actually re-moisturizers -- do prevent some water loss from the skin cells. They cannot, however, deliver life-giving oxygen to the cells. Moisture and other nutrients alone solve only half of the problem. Oxygen is the key. Increase the oxygen level in the cells and you may enhance the cells' ability to metabolize (utilize) all other nutrients.

In a recent study published in the International Journal of Cosmetic Science (Vol. 18, Issue) titled "The Effectiveness of Molecular Oxygen in Cosmetic Formulations", the researchers found that oxygen bound to the oxygen carrrier perfluorodecalin, did indeed increase the oxygen partial pressure as well as the moisture content of the skin. They wrote:

"...this investigation showed that perfluorodecalin plus molecular oxygen improves the barrier function of the skin"

In the last five years, a number of major cosmetic companies, including Lancaster, one of the world's largest, has recognized the importance of oxygen to healthy looking skin. Most of these companies use hydrogen peroxide as an ingredient in their cosmetic lines as the oxygen delivery system. Some have even claimed that they have somehow developed a new way of "stabilizing" the hydrogen peroxide in their creams and gels.

Pure hydrogen peroxide's chemical and electrical nature is very unstable. Sunlight (ultraviolet rays) and heat will break apart this oxygen-rich molecule very easily. Thus, as a cosmetic "ingredient", hydrogen peroxide has a major drawback. Instead of hydrogen peroxide, some smaller "leading edge" companies are now using liquid dissolved oxygen dietary supplements (stabilized oxygen) as their oxygen delivery systems. These oxygen-rich liquids are much more stable and closer to the pH of the skin.

One company combined colostrum with its stabilized oxygen (in a patent pending formula) in its line of cosmetics. We have also seen a remarkable oxygen gel that, upon our initial review, is a wonder skin moisturizer and may prove to be an extremely fine product to improve skin tone while enhancing skin health.

Another company's has emulsified lotions and creams containing stabilized oxygen which are extremely unique. They are designed to allow both oxygen and colostrum to be absorbed into the skin along with the other natural ingredients in the product formulations. The oxygen is immediately dissolved in the extracellular water and in the capillary plasma. As the oxygen penetrates the skin, the oxygen also acts as a vehicle to carry the other ingredients with it, including water.

This transfer of oxygen to the capillaries has been described as a massage to the outer layers of the skin with the claim that epidermal capillaries may become unblocked allowing blood to carry the vital nutrients and oxygen to the cells without hindrance. This results, supposedly, in healthier, more youthful, supple and soft skin with less wrinkles and "character" lines.

For many years, companies like Procter and Gamble® have promoted products featuring hydrogen peroxide (oxygen) in their mouth rinses, tooth pastes and tooth gels. Some companies have also advertised products containing baking soda which is sodium bicarbonate. (It's the oxygen in baking soda that actually does the cleaning, cleansing and disinfecting!) You see, most dental products companies know that oxygen, in one form or another, has remarkable disinfecting, deodorizing and whitening properties.

Current research we've seen by one independent laboratory indicates that stabilized oxygen has clinical tooth whitening abilities. In addition, unlike other whitening products made from hydrogen peroxide or sodium chlorite (chlorine dioxide), these whiteners are not only stable but gentle and totally non-toxic. (Many people complain of tooth sensitivity when using peroxide-based whiteners. Not so with this new generation of whiteners using the newer forms of stabilized oxygen.)

In the next few years, look for oxygen to be a key component in both cosmetic and dental products from companies throughout the world. What was once just a unique "marketing gimmick" is slowly becomming a more established, accepted and important component in product formulations.

Appendix III:

Oxygenated Bottled Water

"All across the planet there is evidence of pollution in rivers, lakes and oceans due to decades of toxic dumping and other such abuses. There is now not a single body of water on the planet which is not affected by pollution."

Energy Times, 1996 Editorial

Early in 1998, the American public heard about a bottled water containing oxygen from the mass media. This was the first time television and newspapers throughout the country embraced the concept of oxygen possibly enhancing athletic performance. Responsible for the media blitz was a fledgling public company out of Florida called Life O2 that touted a patented process that executives of the company called Super-Oxygenation™.

The idea of adding additional oxygen to water is, of course, nothing new. Stabilized oxygen supplements were designed to accomplish this very purpose. Actually, the first oxygenated bottled water, though no longer available, was released back in 1994 by Aquagen International, Inc. called "Aquagen® Artesian Spring Water with Stabilized Oxygen". Aquagen® added its own stabilized oxygen to its bottled water and early literature from the company discussed how this added oxygen could enhance energy. Aquagen® distributed its water through health and nutrition distributors in the U.S.

Why did the media embrace Life O2's new product? To understand this endorsement, we need to grasp the importance and the influence that the bottled water industry maintains over the American -- and for that matter, the world's -- population. At the heart is the growing awareness of the fact that our water supplies are contaminated.

Since the early 1990s, Americans have been acutely aware that their tap water was dangerously polluted with chemicals and dangerous microbes. As early as 1993, a waterborne outbreak of the parasite Cryptosporidium in Milwaukee, Wisconsin, infected an estimated 400,000 residents with flu-like symptoms and killed more than 100 people. That same year a Washington, D.C. water system failed and caused tens of thousands to suffer from diarrhea.

In May of 1994, another outbreak of the same Cryptosporidium parasite killed 19 and sickened more than 100 people in Las Vegas, NV. In fact, a recent survey of water utilities around the country found Cryptosporidium in more than 80 percent of the rivers and lakes that supply 66 major water systems nationwide. (The E.P.A. does not require testing for this organisms!)

Compounding the increase of infectious pathogenic microbes in our water supplies is the significant

TAP WATER'S TOLL

The number of cases of waterborne diseases reported to the Federal Centers for Disease Control and Prevention between 1986 and 1994. During these years, a total of 116 recorded outbreaks struck more than 450,000 individuals. The actual number of cases are certainly higher because the incidents that involve diarrhea, vomiting and nausea are are usually mistaken for the flu.

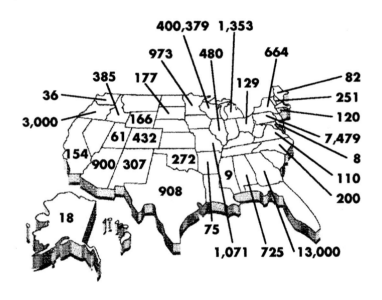

SOURCE: Sierra (July/August 1995)

increase of toxic chemicals in this same supply, exacerbated by the presence of chlorine. Chlorine, used for decades as a water purifier and disinfectant to kill dangerous bacteria like E. coli and deadly parasites with names like Giardia lamblia, Entamoeba coli, Endolimax nana, Blastocystis hominus, entamoeba histolytica and Cryptosporidium, reacts with organic contamination in our water supply to form trihalomethanes (THMs).

Sadly, THMs have been found to cause cancer. Studies of cancer patients around the country suggest that bladder cancer was 220% more frequent in individuals whose water was chlorinated. In fact, some estimates are that chlorine attributes to as many as 10,000 rectal and bladder cancers each year and may be linked to pancreatic cancer and birth defects. **1, 4**

Remember that the term "pathogenic microorganism" represents a class of organisms that cause diseases in plants, animals and humans. This group includes algae, bacteria, viruses and protozoans. They enter our drinking water from human sewage and/or animal feces and cause diseases like dysentery, hepatitis, diariasis, cryptosporidiosis, typhoid fever and cholera. They sicken over 940,000 people a year in the United States and kill as many as 900, usually those with poor resistance to disease including the very old, the very young and those with immune system disorders.

According to one recent report, contaminated water coupled with poor sanitation accounts for over 30,000 deaths each day around the world. That's the equivalent of 100 giant jet liners crashing every day! In fact, in developing nations, 80 percent of the reported diseases affecting human populations are water-related.

Adding to the water quality problem has been the overuse of pesticides by the agricultural industry, organic contamination caused by industry and the massive flooding we have seen throughout the country and the world. This flooding has spread the carcinogenic pesticides from farming lands to the world's water supplies. Flooding is also the contributing factor to the spread of infectious diseases as sewage systems fail!

Recent statistics indicate that more than 3.5 million people in 121 Midwestern cities in the U.S. face an elevated risk of cancer as a result of farm pesticides in drinking water supplies. In fact, one statistic cites that over 14 million Americans routinely consume the weed killers atrazine, cynazine, alachlor, metolachor and simazine. **5**

The worst contaminates in these categories include fertilizers, pesticides, herbicides, paints, fuels, plastics, dyes and preservatives. Each year the chemical industry adds over 10,000 new chemicals to its arsenal of over 10 million formulations. 100,000 of these are used commercially every day around the world. Here's some examples of the danger that pollutants pose to our drinking water: just one gram of a popular household herbicide "2.4-D" can contaminate 10,000,000 liters of drinking water; one drop of common automotive oil can contaminate 25 liters of water; only one gram of PCBs can make up to one billion liters of water unsuitable for freshwater aquatic life.

Finally, even the delivery system that brings water to our homes adds more toxins to our body including copper, lead and radon. In 1993, the U.S. Environmental Protection Agency announced that of 8,100 municipal water systems it tested around the country, 819 residential systems serving more than 30 million Americans were found to have unsafe levels of lead and that 20 percent of all lead contamination is found in drinking water. The symptoms of lead poisoning include nervousness, irritability, headaches, fatigue, musculature problems, constipation and indigestion.

Chronic lead poisoning has been associated with physical, mental and emotional disorders, immune dysfunction, disruption of blood formation, hearing loss, kidney damage and even insanity. Other carcinogenic toxic metals and chemicals in water include arsenic, asbestos, cadmium and cyanides.

Why are we even discussing water? It is because water is so critical to a healthy body. A high percentage of all living organisms, both plant and animal, contains between 70 to 90 percent water. The human body is composed of 75 percent water and the brain contains over 85 percent. As Dr. F. Batmanghelidi, M.D. explains in his excellent book *Your Body's Many Cries for Water*,

"The chemical reactions in all plants and animals that support life take place in a water medium. Water not only provides the medium to make these life sustaining reactions possible, but water itself an important reactant or product of these reactions. In short, the chemistry of life is water chemistry.

"On land, the greatest threat to life is desiccation. Water is lost by evaporation from respiratory surfaces, by evaporation from the body surface, by elimination of feces and by excretion of urine. Lost water must be replaced if life is to continue. It is replaced by drinking, by eating foods containing water and by oxidation of nutrients (water is one of the products of cell metabolism.)" **2**

Just how critical is the regulation of water in our bodies? Even a slight percentage reduction can cause dehydration. In children, the reduction of even a small percentage can become life threatening. As explained by senior medical research specialist Lynn Perentini:

"Without the proper amount of water flushing through our bodies each day, it could trigger a domino effect that contributes to a whole host of problems. When your body is in an extreme state of dehydration, this interferes with the way in which the kidneys purify and remove toxins fro our system. In turn, electrolytes (electrical impulses) are thrown off balance causing us to be unable to perspire, making it difficult for our bodies to retain a constant 98.6 degree body temperature. Without proper perspiration, toxins are also able to accumulate in the body. Just like the concept of 'trickle down economics,' lack of water can have a trickle down effect..." **3**

The two main sources of water sources on the planet are surface water -- from lakes, streams, etc. -- and ground water -- from wells, springs and underground rivers and lakes. Surface water is particularly vulnerable to chemical and micro-organism contamination. Ground water is better protected from micro organisms since the soil and rocks can act as a filter for many of the larger organisms. Yet some organisms do get through to deep water reserves as do many chemical toxins. As Scott Alan Lewis summarized in his article in *Sierra:*

"Here in the United States we assume that our modern technology and scientific knowledge keep those contaminates out of our drinking water. In fact, the American government made that very promise to the American people when it passed the Safe Drinking Water Act in 1974. It strengthened the same law in 1986, and, through the EPA, has set maximum contaminate levels for 84 dangerous substances and pathogens.

"Yet, 20 years after the passage of the law, safe drinking water remains a promise yet to be fulfilled. Some of the contaminate standards set by the EPA are far too weak -- weaker than those in other developed countries. Rules for many dangerous pollutants are still being phased in; some poisons are not regulated at all. Among the latter are certain synthetic organic compounds, radioactive materials, heavy metals, pathogens, and the toxic byproducts created by chlorination or other disinfection techniques." **4**

Because of the very real water quality problem. more and more individuals are turning to bottled water in an attempt to eliminate contamination problems. This is reflected in the tremendous growth -- almost 15 percent per year in the U.S. alone -- of the bottled water industry over the last five years. Americans already consume over 2.7 billion gallons (19.5 gallons per capita) of bottled water making the industry worth over three and a half billion dollars.

Unfortunately, many bottled water companies have been misleading the public for years. According to government statistics (U.S. House Energy and Commerce Commission), as far back as 1991, over one fourth of all bottled water comes from the same sources as the tap water we drink and so contains the same chemical and microorganism contamination.

While this water is supposed to be processed in some manner to reduce these contaminates, estimates are that another fourth of the bottled water on store shelves and delivered to homes and business comes from companies and distributors that cannot provide documentation for the source of their water. In addition, over one third of all bottled water exceeds microbial contamination levels already established by the federal government!

Bottled water is usually described by its source, like spring, spa, geyser, public water supply, etc., by its mineral content, or by the system of treatment it has gone through, like purified, deionized, floridated, steam distilled, ozonated, etc.

NATURAL WATER: This is water from a well, spring or other source where the mineral content is not changed during the bottling process.

SPRING WATER: This is ground water that flows unassisted to a surface opening. Some spring water may be processed prior to bottling, but "natural spring water" generally means that it is unprocessed.

MINERAL WATER: Mineral water contains dissolved minerals. "Natural mineral water" generally contains only minerals found in the water source. This water If a label merely states that it is "mineral water", the chances are that the minerals in the bottled water have been altered, treated or added. Mineral water usually contains a minimum of 500 parts per million (p.p.m.) of total dissolved solids (minerals).

SPARKLING WATER: This is water that is carbonated with carbon dioxide. This gas can be naturally present in the water or it can be added during the bottling process.

NATURALLY CARBONATED MINERAL WATER: This is water usually from geothermic regions that contains high amounts of minerals and naturally occurring dissolved carbon dioxide.

PROCESSED WATER: This is artificially carbonated and filtered waters. Club sodas and seltzers are examples.

R.O. (reverse osmosis) AND DISTILLED WATERS (sometimes called "PURIFIED"): These are waters either processed through specialized filters to remove minerals and other organic contaminates (reverse osmosis) or water that has been boiled producing steam which is then condensed and so contains no minerals or organic contaminates (distilled).

With the rise in bottled water sales has also been a growing demand for healthier and more specialized waters. This consumer interest has sparked the imagination of a small number of bottlers, primarily in the U.S., to add life giving oxygen to their water. Standard bottled water contains varying amounts of dissolved oxygen (O_2) from as little as less than one p.p.m. to perhaps as much as two to three p.p.m. For the most part, don't expect to find much, if any, bioavailable oxygen in any brand of water you buy off the shelf today.

Specialized oxygen-enriched bottled waters come in two basic categories which refer to the method by which oxygen is added to the water: chemical or supplemental additives, including chlorine dioxide, hydrogen peroxide and other stabilized oxygen supplements, and gaseous oxygen.

We've already discussed the many benefits ot adding oxygen supplements to water. But I would like to take a moment to discuss one of the newer techniques using medical grade oxygen as the source of dissolved oxygen in bottled water. Adding gasses to liquid drinks is nothing new. Carbon dioxide gas has been used for decades to add a sparking and refreshing affect to soft drinks, sodas and seltzers. Medical grade oxygen, injected into water under pressure should theoretically be an ideal way to super-saturate water.

Unfortunately, it does have some physical drawbacks. Oxygen added to a liquid under pressure has a more difficult time dissolving in a liquid than does carbon dioxide. As soon as the pressure is released, the oxygen will seek a homeostatic balance and will escape quite rapidly, generally in about 10-20 minutes. The colder the liquid is, the longer the oxygen will take to dissipate.

Also, PET (plastic) bottles, like the ones used for bottled water, are not completely "solid". Though they may look hard like glass, there are tiny spaces between the molecules comprising the plastic where air molecules can escape over time. This reduces the shelf life of bottled water containing oxygen gas. We've heard reports that after two to four weeks, most of the oxygen in these bottles has been significantly reduced.

However, no matter which type of oxygenated water you purchase, any supplemental amount of oxygen you can provide to your body will be beneficial.

FOOTNOTES:

1 AP Release, Telegram Tribune, April 26, 1994.

2 Batmanghelidj, F., M.D. Your Body's Many Cries for Water. p. 1

3 Perentini, Lynn J. Energy Times, Nov/Dec 1996. pp. 43-48.

4 Lewis, Scott Alan. If we're so technologically advanced, why can't we safely drink from our faucets? Sierra. July/August 1995. pp. 55-59.

5 "Millions drink pesticides in water." AP Release, Telegram Tribune, October 18, 1994.

Appendix V:

Oxygen Radicals: A Commonsense Look at Their Nature and Medical Importance
Dr. B. Halliwell, Ph.D.

From the Department of Biochemistry, University of London King's College, London, U.K. Medical Biology 62:71-77, 1984, Rev. 1997

Introduction:

"Oxygen radicals" are now popular subjects for research papers; several hundred are published each year. Many of these pass rapidly into oblivion, joining the great mass of unread scientific literature that clogs library shelves and dilutes important research findings to an increasingly great extent. The basic chemistry of oxygen-derived species was established years ago by radiation chemists (1,6), but "superoxide" is still endowed with miraculous properties by the uninitiated.

Demonstration that the action of a disease or toxin in vivo produces increased lipid peroxidation (a currently-popular scientific activity) means nothing more than the fact that its action produces increased lipid peroxidation: it does not automatically follow that the lipid peroxidation causes the damaging effects of the drug or disease. The purpose of this paper is to explain:

i) what oxygen radicals are;

ii) the evidence that oxygen radicals are important in vivo;

iii) what needs to be done to establish a role for oxygen radicals and lipid peroxidation in human disease.

What are the oxygen radicals and how are they produced?

Electrons within atoms and molecules occupy regions of space known as "orbitals". Each orbital can hold a maximum of two electrons. A single electron alone in an orbital is said to be "unpaired" and a radical is defined as any species that contains one or more unpaired electrons. Such a definition embraces the atom of hydrogen (one unpaired electron) and the ions of such transition metals as iron, copper and manganese (cf. Holmberg, this volume).

The diatomic oxygen molecule, O2, has two unpaired electrons and thus qualifies as a radical. Most of the oxygen taken up by human cells is reduced to water by the action of the cytochrome oxidase complex in mitochondria. This requires the addition of four electrons to each oxygen molecule,

$$O_2 + 4H^+ + 4e^- \longrightarrow 2H_2O \qquad (1)$$

For chemical reasons (reviewed in ref. 21 and 28), O2 likes to receive its electrons one at a time, producing a series of partially reduced intermediates

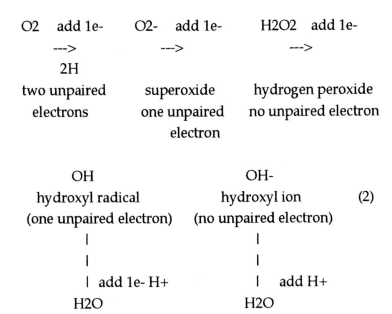

O2   add 1e- O2-   add 1e- H2O2   add 1e-
  --->   --->   --->
  2H

two unpaired superoxide hydrogen peroxide
electrons   one unpaired no unpaired electron
      electron

  OH   OH-
 hydroxyl radical   hydroxyl ion   (2)
(one unpaired electron) (no unpaired electron)
   | |
   | |
  | add 1e- H+ | add H+
 H2O   H2O

Cytochrome oxidase keeps the partially reduced inter-mediates on the pathway to water tightly bound to its active site (21); they do not escape into free solution.

Superoxide: Superoxide ion is the one-electron reduction product of oxygen. Dissolved in organic solvents, it is an extremely reactive species, e.g. it can displace chlorine from such unreactive chlorinated hydrocarbons as carbon tetrachloride (CCl4) (40). In aqueous solution O2- is poorly reactive, acting as a reducing agent (e.g. it will reduce cytochrome C or nitro-blue tetrazolium) and slowly undergoing the dismutation reaction, in which one molecule of superoxide reduces another one to form hydrogen peroxide (H2O2). The dismutation reaction occurs in stages; O2- must first combine with a proton to yield the hydroperoxyl radical, HO2,

$$O_2^- + H^+ \longrightarrow HO_2 \qquad (3)$$
$$HO_2 + O_2 + H^+ \longrightarrow H_2O_2 + O_2 \quad (4)$$
$$\text{overall} \quad O_2^- + O_2^- + 2H^+ \longrightarrow H_2O_2 + O_2 \quad (5)$$

At physiological pH the low concentration of H^+ ions slows the rate of dismutation. Despite the low reactivity of O_2^- in aqueous solution, systems producing it do a great deal of damage in vitro (e.g. they fragment DNA and polysaccharides, kill bacteria and animal cells in culture) and in vivo (e.g. when O_2^- generating systems are injected into the footpads of rats inflammation is produced, their instillation into the lungs of rats and rabbits produces oedema and cell death, and infusion of them into vascular beds produces endothelial cell damage and extensive leakage from the blood vessels) (21,26,28). Depending on the circumstances, damage caused by O_2^- generating systems might be attributed to:

(i) O_2^- itself, e.g. exposure of tissue fluids to O_2^- causes formation of a factor chemotactic for neutrophils that brings more of them into the area and hence can potentiate inflammation;

(ii) HO_2 radical, which is more reactive than O_2^- (6). Formation of HO_2 is favoured at pH values lower than "physiological", but the phagocytic vacuole operates at an acid pH and the pericellular pH of macrophages has been reported to be 6 or less (15);

(iii) H_2O_2 (see below);

(iv) hydroxyl radical (see below);

(v) singlet oxygen. Singlet O_2 is an especially reactive form of oxygen capable of rapidly oxidising many molecules, including membrane lipids. Its formation in O_2--

generating systems has often been proposed but clear-cut evidence for a damaging role of singlet O2 in such systems has not been obtained. One of the problems is that the "scavengers" of singlet O2 frequently used react with other radical species as well (for reviews see ref. 26 and 28).

What is the evidence that O2- is formed in vivo in human cells? Any electron transport chain operating in the presence of O2 "leaks" some of the electrons, passing them directly onto O2. Since O2 prefers to take electrons one at a time, O2- is produced. Such O2- production can be demonstrated in vitro using mitochondria and microsomes from a range of animal tissues. The rate at which O2- is produced rises as the concentration of O2 in the system is raised (e.g. see ref. 20). A number of compounds slowly become oxidised on exposure to O2 and O2- is generated; these include adrenalin, tetrahydrofolate, reduced FMN and oxyhaemoglobin (21, 24).

Since human cells contain mitochondria, endoplasmic reticulum, oxidisable compounds and oxygen, it is likely that O2- is formed within them in vivo. Backing up this evidence, for those who do not like extrapolating from in vitro experiments, is the fact that human cells contain high levels of superoxide dismutase (SOD) activity (45). This enzyme, for which O2- is the specific substrate (35), is known to be a very important anti-oxidant in bacteria and small mammals (26) and its presence in human cells is good evidence that O2- is formed in vivo. During the maturation of erythrocytes most enzymes are lost, but SOD remains. It is not a great stretch of the imagination to associate this with the ability of oxyhaemoglobin to release O2-radical and methaemoglobin.

Another source of O2- in vivo is the respiratory burst of phagocytic cells such as neutrophils, monocytes, eosinophils and macrophages (3, 16, 25). The amount of O2- produced might sometimes be controlled by the O2 tension of body fluids (14). Host defence against invading bacteria is dependent on the circulating neutrophils, which respond to contact with particles they recognise as foreign by producing a "burst" of O2 radical. The particle is engulfed (the piece of membrane surrounding it being the segment that produces O2- on contact; cf. Segal, this volume), and other vesicles then fuse with the phagocytic vesicle. This exposes the engulfed particle to other anti- bacterial mechanisms, including cationic proteins, lysosomal enzymes and myeloperoxidase (3, 16, 25).

Which of these processes is the most important in bacterial killing? Human and other animal neutrophils can kill some strains of bacteria under anaerobic conditions, when O2- cannot form. Obviously, the other mechanisms are important here. Many other bacterial strains are not killed in the absence of O2, however, even though engulfment and vesicle fusion proceed normally. In chronic granulomatous disease (CGD), an inborn error of metabolism, the respiratory burst does not occur but other aspects of phagocytic action proceed normally. CGD was first described in humans because it is accompanied by severe and recurrent infections affecting lymph nodes, skin, lungs and liver (43). The symptoms of CGD provide direct evidence for the production of O2- by human phagocytic cells in vivo and for its role in bacterial killing.

It follows therefore that if neutrophils become activated in the wrong place, or to excessive extents (as in the autoimmune diseases, (25) then the oxygen radicals they release could do a lot of damage. It must be remembered, however, that phagocytic cells also produce hydrolytic enzymes (elastase, neutral proteases etc.), chemotactic factors, prostaglandins, leukotrienes and other chemicals, so that damage by activated phagocytes could be due to any one of these factors or to any combination of them. It cannot be attributed a priori to oxygen radicals.

Hydrogen Peroxide: O_2- generating systems produce H_2O_2 by the dismutation reaction (eqn. 5) and a number of oxidase enzymes produce H_2O_2 directly, examples being glycollate oxidase and amino acid oxidases. SOD enzymes remove O_2- by greatly accelerating the dismutation reaction, so if we accept that O_2- is formed in vivo in humans then we must accept that H_2O_2 vapour is present in expired human breath (48), a likely source being H_2O_2 released from alveolar macrophages (3, 25) although a contribution from peroxide-producing oral bacteria (10) cannot be ruled out.

That H_2O_2 is formed in vivo in humans is further supported by the presence of enzymes specific for its removal, such as catalase and glutathione peroxidase. The latter enzyme requires selenium for its activity (13; cf. Diplock, this volume). H_2O_2 is probably more damaging than is O_2- in in vitro experiments in aqueous solution, but many cells seem to tolerate its presence and bacteria often produce H_2O_2 (e.g. ref. 10). On the other hand, the toxicity of O_2-generating systems to several animal cells in culture has been attributed to formation of H2O2 (e.g. ref. 44). Why this should be so is discussed in the next section.

Hydroxyl radical: Hydroxyl radical is produced when water is exposed to high-energy ionising radiation and hence its properties have been well documented by radiation chemists (6, 49). Unlike the hydroxyl ion, the hydroxyl radical is fearsomely reactive, combining with most molecules found in vivo at near diffusion-controlled rates. Hence any OH produced in vivo will react at or close to its site of formation. The extent of the damage done would therefore depend on what the site of formation was (e.g. production of OH close to DNA could lead to strand breakage whereas production close to an enzyme molecule already present in excess in the cell, such as lactate dehydrogenase, might have no biological consequences).

Hydroxyl radical is produced whenever H2O2 comes into contact with copper (I) ions (Cu+) or iron (II) ions (Fe2+). Dr. Gutteridge has reviewed in this volume the substantial evidence that metal complexes capable of causing hydroxyl radical formation are present in vivo in human cells (also see ref. 28). Particularly important in vivo are complexes of iron salts with phosphate esters such as ATP and GTP (17, 19) or with DNA (18). Organisms take great care to ensure that as much iron or copper as possible is bound to transport proteins or functional proteins such as transferrin, caeruloplasmin or haemoglobin. Metals bound to these proteins are inactive or only weakly active in catalysing OH production (28, 50).

Since both H2O2 and metal complexes are present in vivo in humans, it is logical to assume that OH radicals can form. Direct evidence for this is difficult to obtain. Many methods exist for demonstrating the existence of OH in vitro (see ref. 24 and 28 for reviews) but in vivo any OH formed is likely to react so close to its site of formation that the use of these methods is impractical, although some new techniques (such as the ability of OH to convert dimethylsulphoxide into methane (36) or its ability to hydroxylate aromatic rings in characteristic ways (37) show promise for in vivo use. One can also attempt to infer the formation of OH radical in vivo by observing the damage done (as in rheumatoid arthritis, see below). In vitro, phagocytic cells have been shown to produce OH radical (11-13) and the killing of bacteria can sometimes be prevented by reagents that react with this species (3, 16, 25).

It was mentioned in the previous section that the killing of animal cells in culture by O2- generating systems can sometimes be attributed to H2O2. It could, of course, be achieved by H2O2 itself; some enzymes are known to be inactivated by H2O2 although the best examples come from plant rather than animal systems (11). There is another possibility, however, H2O2 generated externally crosses cell membranes easily and could penetrate inside the cell and cause OH to be formed. Externally added scavengers of OH would not prevent this since they could not reach the correct place. By contrast, O2- crosses cell membranes only slowly (42) unless there is a specific channel for it (the only known example of this being the erythrocyte membrane, which has an "anion channel" through which O2- can move(3). Hydroxyl radical will never cross a membrane: it will react with whatever membrane component if meets first.

What is lipid peroxidation and is it of medical importance? Lipid peroxidation has been broadly defined by A. L. Tappel in the USA as "oxidative deterioration of polyunsaturated fatty acids", i.e. fatty acids that contain more than two carbon-carbon double bonds. Oxygen-dependent deterioration, leading to rancidity, has been long recognised as a problem in the storage of fats and oils and is even more relevant today with the popularity of "polyunsaturated" food products. Some of the best studies on peroxidation chemistry have been carried out by foodchemists.

Initiation of peroxidation in a membrane or polyunsaturated fatty acid is due to the attack of any species that can "pull off" a hydrogen atom from one of the - CH_2 - groups in the carbon chain. Hydroxyl radical and possibly HO_2 can do this, but H_2O_2 and O_2- cannot. Hence O_2- does not initiate lipid peroxidation. Since a hydrogen atom has only one electron, removing it leaves behind an unpaired electron on the carbon. The resulting carbon radical - CH -, undergoes molecular rearrangement to form a conjugated diene, which then combines rapidly with O_2 to give a peroxy radical.

$$O_2$$
$$|$$
$$- CH -$$

Peroxy radicals are capable of abstracting a hydrogen atom from other fatty acids and so setting off a chain reaction that can continue until the membrane fatty acids are completely oxidised to hydroperoxides (eqn. 6)

$$O_2$$
$$|$$

- CH -   +   - CH2 -   --->
peroxy   adjacent fatty acid
radical   carbon chain

$$O_2H$$

- CH -   +   - CH -   (6)
carbon radical,   lipid
forms another   hydroperoxide
peroxy radical

Lipid hydroperoxides are stable under physiological conditions until they come into contact with transition metals such as iron or copper salts. Cu^{2+}, Fe^{2+} or Fe^{3+} salts as well as haem and haem proteins (e.g. cytochromes, haemoglobin) can interact with lipid peroxides. These metals or their complexes cause lipid hydroperoxides to decompose in very complicated ways, producing radicals that can continue the chain reaction of lipid peroxidation (as in eqn. 6), as well as cytotoxic aldehydes and hydrocarbon gases. Most attention is paid in the literature to malonaldehyde, but this is a very minor endproduct of lipid peroxidation (for reviews see ref. 4, 26, 32).

Does lipid peroxidation occur normally in vivo in humans? This question is surprisingly difficult to answer: little evidence for lipid peroxides or their decomposition products can be found in healthy human tissues (28). Expired human breath contains gaseous hydrocarbons that might have originated from decomposition of lipid hydroperoxides, but they might also have been produced by bacteria in the gut or even on the skin. Animal cell membranes contain tocopherol (vitamin E), which is a powerful inhibitor of lipid peroxidation, and proteins such as caeruloplasmin and glutathione peroxidase probably help to protect against this process in vivo (27).

Diseased tissues, or tissues isolated after exposure of animals to such toxins as ethanol, phenylhydrazine and paraquat often show evidence of increased peroxidation. Simple in vitro experiments demonstrate quite clearly that dead or damaged tissues peroxidise more rapidly than living ones, presumably because of membrane disruption by enzymes released from lysosomes, release of metal ions from their storage sites and failure of antioxidant mechanisms. Thus evidence that a toxin increases lipid peroxidation in vivo does not prove the sequence of events

$$\text{toxin} \longrightarrow \text{lipid peroxidation} \longrightarrow \text{damage} \qquad (7)$$

but is equally explained by the sequence:

$$\text{toxin} \longrightarrow \text{cell damage or death} \longrightarrow \text{lipid peroxidation} \qquad (8)$$

Of course, toxins released by dead or dying cells undergoing peroxidation might cause further damage to healthy cells, although there is little evidence for this in vivo.

Among the many claims I have seen in the literature for lipid peroxidation as an agent of the damage induced by a toxin, I have seen clear evidence for sequence 7 only in the case of the hepatotoxic effects of carbon tetrachloride (32). Sequence 8 is a much better explanation of the in vivo effects on membrane lipids of, for example, paraquat.

An often quoted illustration of the importance of lipid peroxidation in vivo is the accumulation of "age pigment" in various human tissues. Chemical analysis of age pigment shows convincingly that it is an endproduct of oxidative damage to lipids (41). However, the lipids in question seem to be taken into lysosomes before they are degraded; they are not "normal cell lipids". The exposure of lipids to hydrolytic enzymes and metal ions within lysosomes no doubt facilitates their peroxidation, and so more peroxidised material accumulates within cells as lysosomes get older and have engulfed more lipid material.

The TBA test: The TBA (thiobarbituric acid) test is one of the most widely used (and abused!) tests for measuring lipid peroxidation. The simplicity of performing the test (the material under study is merely heated with acid and TBA and the formation of a pink colour measured at 523 nm) conceals its essential complexity.

Consider a typical experiment. A lipid system, perhaps with added metal ions, chelating agents or other reagents, in incubated in the presence of air. Then TBA plus acid are added and the mixture heated at 100 degrees Celsius.

The air, metals and other reagents are still present, so as much or even more oxidative damage to the lipid can be done during the TBA test itself as happened during the initial incubation.

The pink colour is due to the formation of an adduct between TBA and malonaldehyde (MDA) under acidic conditions. Indeed, the TBA assay is often calibrated with MDA and the results of peroxidation assays are often expressed as "amounts of MDA formed". Some papers in the literature give the mistaken impression that TBA reacts only with free MDA and so measures the production, but it was shown as long ago as 1958 in studies with peroxidising fish oil that 98 % of the MDA that reacts in the TBA test was not present in the original sample assayed but forms from lipid peroxides that decomposed during the acid-heating stage of the TBA assay.

More recent studies confirm this and show that the apparent "TBA reactivity" of say, serum, varies with the exact concentration of acid, type of acid and period of heating used in the TBA assay (23). The amount of MDA formed during the initial incubation of the system as opposed to during the assay depends on such factors as the iron salt concentration (4, 23, 32). An apparent "inhibitor" of lipid peroxidation as detected by the TBA test might actually inhibit the peroxidation process, but could equally well interfere with decomposition of the peroxides during the acid-heating stage of the assay. Similarly, absolute values for the "TBA reactivity" of body fluids or tissue extracts are meaningless, although changes in these values may be significant provided that the same assay is employed in the same way each time.

Of course, many scientists are aware of these problems with the TBA assay and there are ways around them

(2, 41), including the use of other assay systems in conjunction with the TBA test (4, 27). I have included these cautions to encourage a more critical attitude to some of the published literature.

Oxygen Radicals and Disease: Free radicals have been suggested to be involved in the pathology of a number of diseases. In several cases the evidence consists only of observations of increased lipid peroxidation in diseased tissues, which is ambiguous (see above). I have chosen to look in detail at two cases where the evidence at first sight is more convincing, cancer and inflammatory joint disease.

Cancer: Any substance that reacts with DNA is potentially carcinogenic. Exposure of DNA to O2- generating systems causes extensive strand breakage and degradation of deoxyribose (9, 39), an effect shown in vitro to be due to formation of OH.

Both bacteria and animal cells in culture suffer DNA damage on exposure to O2- generating systems, which can be shown to be mutagenic (46, 47). It is therefore tempting to attribute the increased risk of development of cancer in chronically inflamed tissues to generation of oxygen radicals by phagocytic cells, although there is no direct evidence for this.

Great excitement was generated by reports that cancer cells in culture and from some transplantable tumours in animals are deficient in SOD activity, especially in their mitochondria (for a review see ref. 34). The relevance of these studies to human cancer is not at all clear, however, since human tumours biopsied during surgery show no defects in any SOD activity (31, 45).

Rheumatoid arthritis: I have already speculated on the role of oxygen radicals in the autoimmune diseases. Rheumatoid arthritis has some of the features of an autoimmune disease but its exact cause is unknown. The synovial fluid of the inflamed joint swarms with neutrophils. Since the fluid contains increased concentrations of products that activated neutrophils release (including lactoferrin, 5) and end-products of arachidonic acid metabolism), then at least some of these neutrophils must be activated and thus producing superoxide, and hence H2O2 in vivo.

Human synovial fluid is poor in SOD, catalase and glutathione peroxidase activities (8) but does contain iron complexes capable of catalyzing a reaction between O2- and H2O2 to form OH (38). There is as yet no direct proof that OH is formed in vivo, but evidence consistent with its formation includes the observation that the hyaluronic acid in synovial fluid is degraded in rheumatoid joints, and the type of degradation observed can be reproduced by exposing pure hyaluronic acid in vitro to OH radical (22).

TBA-reactive material is also present in serum and synovial fluid of rheumatoid patients. There are significant correlations (38) between the content of TBA-reactive material in synovial fluid, its content of catalytic iron complexes and both clinical ("knee score") and laboratory ("white cell count" and "fluid content of C-reactive protein") assessments of disease activity.

Thus there is certainly evidence for oxygen radicals being produced in the rheumatoid joint and having some deleterious effects. The question to be answered is how important are oxygen radicals in relation to other agents of damage. The pathology of rheumatoid arthritis is very complex and the number of potentially damaging agents, including hydrolytic enzymes, prostaglandins and leukotrienes, is enormous (29).

Some scientist have tried to assess the importance of oxygen radicals by examining the effects of injecting SOD directly into inflamed joints (33; see Marklund, this volume), whereas our group, reasoning that iron complexes are required for O2- dependent formation of highly reactive OH radical, is examining the effect of iron-chelating drugs that can prevent OH formation (such as desferrioxamine, 12) on animal models of acute and chronic inflammation (7).

REFERENCES:

1. Anbar M, Neta P: A compilation of specific bimolecular rate constants for the reactions of hydrated electrons, hydrogen atoms and hydroxyl radicals with inorganic and organic compounds in aqueous solution. Int J Appl Radiat Isot 18: 495-523, 1967

2. Aust SD, Svingen BA: The role of iron in enzymatic lipid peroxidation. In: Free radicals in biology, vol. 5. ED. W. A. Pryor. Academic Press, New York 1982

3. Babior BM: Oxygen-dependent microbial killing by phagocytes. N Engl J Med 298: 721-725, 1978

4. Barber AA, Berheim F: Lipid peroxidation: its measurement, occurrence and significance. Adv Gerontol Res 2: 355-403, 1967

5. Bennett RM, Eddie-Quartey AC, Holt PJL: Lactoferrin: an iron binding protein in synovial fluid. Arthritis Rheum 16: 186-190, 1973

6. Bielski BHJ, Shive GG: Reaction rates of superoxide radicals with the essential amino acids. In: Oxygen free radicals and tissue damage. Ciba Found Symp 65 (new series). Excerpta Medica, Amsterdam 1979

7. Blake DR, Hall ND, Bacon PA, Dieppe PA, Halliwell B, Gutteridge JMC: Effect of a specific iron chelating agent on animal models of inflammation. Ann Rheum Dis 42: 89-93, 1983

8. Blake DR, Hall ND, Treby DA, Halliwell B, Gutteridge JMC: Protection against superoxide and hydrogen peroxide in synovial fluid from rheumatoid patients. Clin Sci 61: 483-486, 1981

9. Brawn K, Fridovich I: DNA strand scission by enzymically generated oxygen radicals. Arch Biochem Biophys 206: 414-419, 1981

10. Carlsson J, Iwami Y, Yamada T: H_2O_2 excretion by oral streptococci and effect of lactoperoxidase-thiocyanate-H_2O_2. Infect Immun 40: 70-80, 1983

11. Charles SA, Halliwell B: Effect of H_2O_2 on spinach chloroplast fructose bis phosphatase. Biochem J 189: 373-376, 1980

12. Gutteridge JMC, Richmond R, Halliwell B: Inhibition of the iron-catalysed formation of hydroxyl radicals from superoxide and of lipid peroxidation by desferrioxamine. Biochem J 184: 469-472, 1979

13. Diplock AT: Metabolic and functional defects in selenium deficiency. Phil Trans R Soc Lond B 294: 105-117, 1981

14. Edwards SW, Hallet MD, Lloyd D, Campbell AK: Decrease in apparent Km for oxygen after stimulation of respiration of rat polymorphonuclear leucocytes. FEBS Lett 161: 60-64, 1983

15. Etherington DJ, Silver IA, Gibbons R: An in vitro model for the study of collagen degradation during acute inflammation. Life Sci 25: 1885-1892, 1979

16. Fantone JC, Ward PA: Role of oxygen-derived free radicals and metabolites in leukocyte-dependent inflammatory reactions. Am J Pathol 107: 397-413, 1982

17. Flitter W, Rowley DA, Halliwell B: Superoxide-dependent formation of hydroxyl radicals in the presence of iron salts. What is the physiological iron chelator? FEBS Lett 158: 310-312, 1983

18. Floyd RA: DNA-ferrous iron catalysed hydroxyl free radical formation from hydrogen peroxide. Biochem Biophys Res Commun 99: 1209-1215, 1981

19. Floyd RA: Direct demonstration that ferrous ion complexes of di- and triphosphate nucleotides catalyse hydroxyl free radical formation from hydrogen peroxide. Arch Biochem Biophys 225: 263-270, 1983

20. Freeman, BA, Crapo JD: Hyperoxia increases oxygen radical production in rat lungs and lung mitochondria. J Biol Chem 256: 10986-10992, 1981

21. Fridovich I: Superoxide radical, an endogeneous toxicant. Ann Rev Pharmacol Toxicol 23: 239-257, 1983

22. Greenwald AA, Moy WW: Effect of oxygen-derived free radicals on hyaluronic acid. Arthritis Rheum 23: 455-463, 1980

23. Gutteridge JMC: Free radical damage to lipids, amino acids, carbohydrates and nucleic acids as determined by thiobarbituric acid reactivity. Int J Biochem 14: 649-653, 1982

24. Halliwell B: Free radicals, oxygen toxicity and aging. In: Age pigments. Ed. R. S. Sohal. Elsevier, Amsterdam 1981

25. Halliwell B: Production of superoxide, hydrogen peroxide and hydroxyl radicals by phagocytic cells: a cause of chronic inflammatory disease? Cell Biol Int Rep 6: 529-542, 1982

26. Halliwell B: Superoxide and the superoxide theory of oxygen toxicity: a critical appraisal. In: Copper proteins, vol. 2. Ed. R. Lontie. CRC Press, Florida 1984

27. Halliwell B, Gutteridge JMC: Free radicals in biology and medicine. Oxford University Press, Oxford 1984

28. Halliwell B, Gutteridge JMC: Oxygen toxicity, oxygen radicals, transition metals and disease. Biochem J 219: 1-14, 1984

29. Henderson B: The biochemistry of the human synovial lining with special reference to alterations in metabolism in rheumatoid arthritis. Path Res Pract 172: 1-24, 1981

30. Lynch RE, Fridovich I: Permeation of the erythrocyte stroma by superoxide radical. J Biol Chem 253: 4697-4699, 1978

31. Marklund SL, Westman NG, Lundgren E, Roos G: Copper and zinc- containing SOD, manganese-containing

SOD, catalase and glutathione peroxidase in normal and neoplastic human cell lines and normal human tissues. Cancer Res 42: 1955-1961, 1982

32. McBrien DCH, Slater TF (eds): Free radicals, lipid peroxidation and cancer. Academic Press, London 1982

33. Michelson AM, Puget K: Aspects medicaux des superoxyde dismutases. CR Seances Soc Biol 173: 380-394, 1979

34. Oberley LW: Superoxide dismutase and cancer. In: Superoxide dismutase, vol. 2. Ed. L. W. Oberley. CRC Press, Florida 1982

35. Pain RH: Dressing the SOD. Nature 306: 228, 1983

36. Repine JE, Eaton JW, Anders MW, Hoidal JR, Fox RB: Generation of hydroxyl radical by enzymes, chemicals and human phagocytes in vitro. J Clin Invest 64: 1642-1651, 1979

37. Richmond R, Halliwell B, Chauhan J, Darbre A: Superoxide- dependent formation of hydroxyl radicals: detection of hydroxyl radicals by the hydroxylation of aromatic compounds. Anal Biochem 118: 328-335, 1981

38. Rowley D, Gutteridge JMC, Blake D, Farr M, Halliwell B: Lipid peroxidation in rheumatoid arthritis. Thiobarbituric-acid- reactive material and catalytic iron salts in synovial fluid from rheumatoid patients. Slin Sci (in press) 1984

39. Rowley DA, Halliwell B: DNA damage by superoxide-generating systems in relation to the mechanism of action of the anti- tumour antibiotic adriamycin. Biochim Biophys Acta 761: 86-93, 1983

40. Sawyer DT, Gibian MT: The redox chemistry of superoxide ion. Tetrahedron 35: 1471-1481, 1979

225

41. Sohal RS (ed): Age pigments. Elsevier, Amsterdam 1981

42. Takahashi MA, Asada K: Superoxide anion permeability of phospholipid membranes and chloroplast thylakoids. Arch Biochem Biophys 226: 558-566, 1983

43. Tauber AI, Borregaard N, Simons E, Wright J: Chronic granulomatous disease: a syndrome of phagocyte oxidase deficiencies. Medicine 62: 286-309, 1983

44. Weiss SJ, Young J, LoBuglio AF, Slivka A, Nimeh NF: Role of hydrogen peroxide in neutrophil-mediated destruction of cultured endothelial cells. J Clin Invest 68: 714-721, 1981

45. Westman NG, Marklund SL: Copper-and zinc-containing superoxide dismutase and manganese-containing superoxide dismutase in human tissues and human malignant tumours. Cancer Res 41: 2962-2966, 1981

46. Weitburg AB, Weitzman SA, Destrempes M, Latt SA, Stossel TP: Stimulated human phagocytes produce cytogenetic changes in cultured mammalian cells. N Engl J Med 308: 26-30, 1983

47. Weitzman SA, Stossel TP: Mutation caused by human phagocytes. Science 212: 546-547, 1981

48. Williams MD, Leight JS, Chance B: Hydrogen peroxide in human breath and its probable role in spontaneous breath luminescence. Ann NY Acad Sci 45: 478-483, 1983

49. Willson RL: Free radicals and tissue damage: mechanistic evidence from radiation studies. In: Biochemical mechanism of liver injury. Ed. T. F. Slater. Academic Press, London 1978

50. Winterbourn CC: Lactoferrin-catalysed hydroxyl radical formation. Additional requirement for a chelating agent. Biochem J 210: 15-19, 1983

Author's Address:

Dr. B. Halliwell, Ph.D.
Department of Biochemistry,
University of London
King's College, Strand, London, UK

Appendix V:

HYPER-OXYGENATION

Waves Forest, Publisher
Now What? 1989, rev. 1997

Several dozen AIDS patients have not only reversed their death sentences, but are now back at work, completely free of the disease. They destroyed the virus in their blood by hyper-oxygenation, known in various forms as oxygen therapy, bio-oxidative therapy or autohemotherapy. This is a simple, inexpensive and very broad spectrum process that many feel could force a complete overhaul of the medical industry. The two basic types of oxygen therapy are ozone blood infusion, and absorption of oxygen water (hydrogen peroxide) at very low concentrations.

It turns out that the AIDS virus cannot tolerate high oxygen levels in its victims' blood. Not only that, every other disease organism tested so far has the same weakness. Even cancer growths contract and disappear when the oxygen saturation is sufficiently increased in the fluids surrounding them, since they are anaerobic.

AIDS, herpes, hepatitis, Epstein Barr, cytomegalovirus and other lipid envelope virus are readily destroyed by hyper-oxygenating the patient's blood with ozone. This was demonstrated by among others Dr. Horst Kief in Bad Hersfeld, West Germany. Dr. Kief has already cured a number of AIDS victims by drawing blood, infusing it with ozone and returning it to the patient, at regular intervals until all the virus is gone. (He can be reached through Biozon Ozon-Technik GmbH, An Der Haune #10, Bad Hersfeld, D-6430, Federal Republic of Germany). Dr. S. Rilling of Stuttgart and Dr. Renate Viebahn of Iffezheim are among the growing number of physicians who have obtained similar results with their patients. They are with Arztlich Gesellschaft fur Ozonetherapie and JrJ Hansler GmbH, respectively.

The Basis Of Bio-oxidative Thera-pies:

For many years the health sciences have been seeking to identify the primary physical cause of all diseases, and the cure-all that this basic principal would yield. Now both have been found, but their utter simplicity makes them difficult to accept at first, since it seems like if it's that easy, we should have been using them all along.

Our bodies are composed mostly of water, which is eight ninths oxygen. Most nutritional studies tend to get caught up in the small details of biochemistry and overlook our most abundant and essential element, and the fundamental role of its depletion in causing illness. Of all the elements the body needs, only oxygen is in such constant demand that its absence brings death in minutes.

The main difference, for healing purposes, between benign microorganisms (including our own cells), and those which cause disease, is that the latter require much lower oxygen levels. This is due to their more primitive evolutionary origins, during the ages when free oxygen was far less abundant. Now their descendants can only survive in low oxygen environments such as accompany stagnation and decay. To become a growth medium for such parasites, one has to have allowed the oxygen saturation of the body's fluids to drop well below the optimum level for healthy cell growth and function.

The simplest substances available for restoring one's oxygen balance to a healthy range are ozone (O3), and hydrogen peroxide (H2O2), which is much easier to obtain and use. They are both highly toxic when concentrated, which has tended to obscure their germicidal value except as a skin antiseptic. But when diluted to therapeutic levels (for H2O2, 1/2 of 1% or less), they are not only non-toxic but uniquely beneficial.

Ozone Blood Treatment: Ozone overcomes the AIDS virus by a fundamentally different process than usually attempted by drugs. Instead of burdening the liver and immune system with more elaborate toxic substances, ozone simply oxidizes the molecules in the shell of the virus.

The treatment is remarkably simple. The ozone is produced by forcing oxygen through a metal tube carrying a 300 volt charge. A pint of blood is drawn from the patient and placed in an infusion bottle. The ozone is then forced into the bottle and mixed in by shaking gently, whereupon the blood turns bright cardinal red. As the ozone molecules dissolve into the blood they give up their third oxygen atom, releasing considerable energy which destroys all lipid-envelope virus, and apparently all other disease organisms as well, while leaving blood cells unharmed.

It also oxygenates the blood to a greater degree than is usually reached, what with poor air and sluggish breathing habits. The treated blood is then given back to the patient. This treatment is given from twice a week to twice a day, depending on how advanced the disease is. The strengthened blood confers some of its virucidal properties to the rest of the patient's blood as it disperses. The disease will not return, as long as the patient maintains his blood in an oxygen positive state, through proper breathing, exercise, and clean diet.

Dr. Preuss, in Stuttgart, has written up ten case histories of AIDS patients he has cured by this method. But his and the other physicians' reports are all anecdotal rather than in the form of "controlled studies", since they could not be expected to treat some patients and deny treatment to others just for the purpose of accumulating evidence. Thus their results are not considered "proof" by the US medical community. So the Medizone Company in New York has taken on the task of doing the controlled studies required for the treatment to be approved in the US for general use.

In the summer of 1986 Medizone obtained from the FDA an IND (Investigative New Drug) Approval for ozone, which falls under the heading of drugs even though it isn't. They verified that ozone destroys the AIDS virus in vitro, and completed their animal tests in the fall of 1986. The tests demonstrated no indication of toxicity, at ten times the equivalent amount that is proposed for human treatment.

The Medizone Company is at 123 E 54th St. Suite 2B, NY, NY 10022: phone is 212-421-0303. Medizone says that it has obtained the rights to US patent #4,632,980, on "ozonation of blood and blood products", from the company "Immunologics", in exchange for Medizone stock shares.

The patent pertains specifically to inactivating lipid-envelope virus. In humans, this includes AIDS, herpes, hepatitis, Epstein Barr virus, and cytomegalovirus, among others. Medizone obtained tentative FDA approval in April 1987 to begin human testing, but for a variety of "bureaucratic reasons" the FDA has postponed the actual start of the tests eight times now, with requests for further data, some of which had already been given to them.

Twenty months now have passed [as of December 1988], along with several thousand AIDS victims, since the first announced starting date was postponed. The Medizone staff was hoping to finally begin in the spring of 1989, but are no longer announcing expected starting dates with much confidence. "There are no technical problems, but this is the FDA we're dealing with, after all."

As the Company's future hangs on their decision, no one at Medizone wants to risk antagonizing the FDA, by speculating about their actual motives for stalling such a broad-spectrum cure.

All this can be done with virtually no publicity. The official reason for it is that the accepted procedure for publishing medical breakthroughs is to complete all the tests first, even though victims may die waiting for the cautious, methodical testing procedure to run its course. No one in the industry wants to raise false hopes, let alone repeat the medical disasters that have resulted in the past, from rushing approval on new treatments.

On the other hand, the enormously expensive and dubiously effective drug AZT was widely publicized and many months before it was approved in the US, as is ongoing research into possible AIDS vaccines. In fact, FDA

Commissioner Frank Young has even announced a proposal to make experimental drugs available to AIDS victims as swiftly as possible, without waiting for full FDA approval procedure to be completed. So there appears to be a severe double standard involved here.

It seems that highly profitable "treatments" with serious side effects can be promoted through massive news coverage, while an actual cure, repeatedly demonstrated in Europe, with minimal cost and no apparent harmful effects, must be delayed and kept quiet while panic and deaths mount. Surely at this stage the benefits of unauthorized publicity will outweigh the risks.

Safe Purification Of Blood For Transfusions: Ozone infusion also provides a simple method of purifying stored blood and blood components, eliminating any possibility of disease being transmitted by transfusion. It also pre-oxygenates blood to be transfused, greatly reducing the burden on the body receiving the blood.

This application alone, of the Medizone process has enormous profit potential, and the treatment will have vast international demand as the news spreads. This has not gone unnoticed by various investment analysts. "Confidential: report from Zurich", "Penny Stock Insider" and "Low-Priced Stock Edition", among others, are urging their readers to get in on Medizone now, comparing the opportunity to getting in on Xerox, IBM, or Polaroid when they were still unknown.

Various physicians have independently discovered ozone to be also effective against cancer, leukemia, arthritis, coronary heart disease, arterial circulation disorders. colitis, gum diseases, and assorted childrens' diseases. Some of these findings have now been collected and published in the volume, "Medical Applications of Ozone", available from the International Ozone Association, 83 Oakwood Terrace, Norwalk, CT 06850.

Some of the medical uses of ozone have been appreciated for years in Europe, Brazil, and elsewhere, as well as its advantages over chlorine for water treatment (no toxic residues, 5,000 times more rapid disinfection) but its still relatively unknown in the US.

Oxygen Water: A much simpler type of Oxygen Therapy uses hydrogen peroxide (H_2O_2) which is what ozone (O_3) forms on contact with water. It can be taken orally if diluted with water to 1/200 or less, absorbed through the skin by bathing in it (anywhere from 1-8 pints of 3% H_2O_2 in a standard size bathtub half full), or in severe cases it can be injected (250 cc of .075% to .15% or roughly 1/1300 to 1/650). Injections obviously require a physicians assistance, but self treatment is possible with oral and skin applications.

The principle is the same as with ozone blood treatment. All hostile micro-organisms prefer lower oxygen levels than the body's cells require to remain healthy. Boosting the oxygen level revitalizes normal cells while killing viruses and other pathogens.

The domestic sales of hydrogen peroxide are rising at 15% per year, as the news of this option spreads at the grass roots level. The rapid expansion of the peroxide movement is especially remarkable considering there has been almost no media coverage, and in fact the FDA, American Cancer Society and other enforcers of established medicine have tried hard to discourage the practice. Hydrogen peroxide is the only germicidal agent composed only of water and oxygen. Like ozone, it kills disease organisms by oxidation as it spreads through the patient's tissues.

This also destroys cancerous growths which are anaerobic. Nobel prize winner Dr. Otto Warburg demonstrated over 50 years ago the basic difference between normal cells and cancer cells. Both derive energy from glucose, but the normal cell requires oxygen to combine with the glucose, while cancer cells break down glucose without oxygen, yielding only 1/15 the energy per glucose molecule that a normal cell produces. This is why cancer cells have such a huge appetite for sugar, and also why people who consume excessive quantities of sugar tend to get cancer more often.

The anaerobic breakdown of glucose by cancer cells forms large amounts of lactic acid as a waste product, the same substance formed by fermentation of lactose, as in spoiled milk. The liver converts some of this back into glucose, in an attempt to salvage a food source from a toxic waste. In doing this the liver uses 1/5 the energy per glucose molecule than a normal cell can derive from it, but that's three times the energy a cancer cell will get from it. The more the weak, deranged cancer cells multiply, the more energy is lost to the normal cells. Thus we find that low levels of both oxygen and energy tend to occur where cancer is present, and vice versa. This wasteful metabolism becomes self-sustaining and dominant unless the oxygen and/or energy levels are sharply increased, or the cancer's food source is eliminated.

Heart Transplant Pioneer Recommends Oxygen Water: Dr. Christian Bernard, who performed the first heart transplant, said in march 1986 that he was taking peroxide and water himself, several times daily to reduce arthritis and aging, and he recommended it highly at the time. Since then he has come under heavy attack by the medical establishment for this position, and now states that he "is not involved" with the peroxide movement. But he does not retract his original endorsement, nor deny that he still uses it personally.

Hundreds of physicians are already curing a broad assortment of "incurables" with this natural anti-microbial agent. This includes some forty or more in the US. A principal liaison to these free-thinking physicians is DR. Charles H. Farr, who wrote "The Therapeutic Use of Intravenous Hydrogen Peroxide". He directs the International Bio-Oxidative Medicine Foundation, and publishes the "IBOM Newsletter" which contains procedural updates and technical refinements for physicians using intravenous H_2O_2 therapy on their patients. By classifying the treatments as experimental they can get around the FDA's archaic restrictions for now, until massive public demand and/or media exposure force official approval.

Dr. Farr summarizes the beneficial effects of H_2O_2 in "IBOM" issue #2; these include killing bacteria, protozoa, yeast, and virus, oxidizing lipids from arterial walls, increasing oxygen tension intracellularly, stimulating oxidative enzymes, returning elasticity to arterial walls, dilating coronary vessels, and regulating membrane transport. Dr. Farr is at 1130 North May Ave, Oklahoma City, OK 73120; 405-752-0070 and 799-8781.

Dr. Kurt W. Donsbach at the Bio-Genesis Institute in Rosarita Beach, Baja Mexico (714-964-1535), has achieved a remission rate exceeding 70% in over 300 patients, at last count, most of whom had been previously told they were beyond hope, and had "tried everything else". Bio-oxidative therapies are now applied to all cases that arrive at this clinic, and all respond except for those who arrive already very close to death. The Guadalahara Medical School, Mexico's largest, is initiating their own tests this summer, and will add it to their curriculum upon verification.

As Dr. Donsbach has pointed out, no U.S. clinic or institution has ever tested intravenous H2O2 as a treatment for cancer, so any claim that it is not effective is not based on clinical trial, and amounts to willful dis-information. The Gerson Institute and La Gloria Clinic in Mexico are also using Hydrogen Peroxide therapies on their patients, after the staff tested it on themselves and found it beneficial.

Hydrogen Peroxide In Nature: Hydrogen peroxide occurs naturally in rain and snow, from atmospheric ozone, and in mountain streams where rushing water is continuously aerated. Most of us learned at an early age to drink from a stream only where the water is running white, because that is where it gets cleansed of germs. The reason is that H2O2 is forming there due to its rapid agitation, and that's what kills any harmful microbes present. By just shaking a bottle of water vigorously for a while you can tuck enough extra oxygen into it to form detectable amounts of H2O2, improving its purity, flavor and vitality.

It turns out that the spring waters at Lourdes, France, long recognized for their remarkable healing properties, are very high in natural hydrogen peroxide. The spring is fed by high altitude snow melt, so the snow apparently absorbs unusually large quantities of ozone on its way from the upper atmosphere. Other less-known high altitude springs are said to be likewise effective.

Similar benefits can be obtained in a swimming pool or hot tub, by discarding the chlorination system and simply pouring in H2O2, or by bubbling ozone through the water. One simple method of making pool-grade ozone is to pump air past an enclosed ultraviolet lamp.

Raw, uncooked vegetables and fruits can contain natural hydrogen peroxide. Cooking drives off the extra oxygen. Fresh fruit juices are well known for their blood cleansing and revitalizing capabilities, particularly when they are not combined with other foods; this is largely due to the H2O2 they contain. Reconstituted frozen juices have much less and are no longer "alive", thus they are not nearly as effective.

H2O2 Is The Heart of The Immune System: Mother's milk contains a high amount of H2O2, especially colostrum, the first milk secreted after birth, which activates the newborn's immune system, and is the key to many other metabolic processes.

Under conditions of optimum health, H2O2 is produced by the body's immune system in whatever amounts are needed to quickly destroy any invading hostile organisms. It is made by combining water in the body with the free oxygen that is supposed to be available.

When the body is oxygen-starved, it can't produce enough H2O2 to wipe out invading pathogens, which can then get the upper hand and cause visible disease.

Oxygen Boost Is Key To Other Healing Methods: When penicillin is effective against infection, it is largely due to the formation of bacterial amounts of H2O2, when glucose is oxidized by O2 in the presence of penicillin notatin. (General Biochemistry, Fruton & Simmonds 577.1 F944 p. 339)

Much has been made about the healing properties of interferon, but it is unbelievably expensive. However, much of its effectiveness is apparently due to the fact that it stimulates the production of H2O2 and other oxygen intermediates, which are a key factor in reactivating the immune system. (Journal of Interferon Research Vol 3, #2, 1983 p. 143-151.) Thus Interferon may turn out to be simply a very elaborate way to accomplish essentially the same thing as H2O2 regimen.

Vitamin C (ascorbic acid) has long been recognized as essential to the proper use of oxygen by the cells. Dr. Linus Pauling has demonstrated that large doses of vitamin C are effective against cancer. The mainstream medical community still has not acknowledged this discovery, let alone put it to use, despite Dr. Pauling's previous credentials.

As it turns out, vitamin C actually creates extra H2O2 in the body.

Organic Germanium (bis-carboxyethyl germanium sesquioxide) is gaining increasing recognition as a potent healing substance, primarily through the work of Dr. Kasuhiko Asai. This compound directly increases the body's oxygen supply, as it contains a great deal of oxygen in a form that can be easily assimilated. (See "Miracle Cure: Organic Germanium" by Dr. Paul Asai, Japan Publications, Inc., Tokyo and New York.)

Taheebo (aka Pau D'Arco or Lapacho Colorado) is a tree that grows in the Andes and fixes high concentrations of oxygen in crystalline form in its inner bark. The bark has been used for centuries by the native peoples of the area to prevent and reverse illness, and it is one reason why they do not get cancer. In recent years it has become popular in the US, and it gets by the FDA as an "herbal tea" whose distributors wisely make no medical claims for it. Again, much of its effectiveness is apparently due to its high oxygen content, released in solution when brewed as a tea.

Causes of Oxygen Depletion: There are several common practices that drop a person's oxygen level far below what it should really be. At sea level, 20% of the atmosphere is supposed to be oxygen, but city air gets down as low as 10%, due to smog and removal of trees. Air that tastes bad induces a tendency to breathe shallowly, getting even less oxygen to the blood. So does lack of exercise.

The carbon monoxide (CO) in smog does not normally occur in nature in much quantity since it's formed by incomplete combustion of carbon compounds. It is electrically unbalanced, so it seeks to bond with any available oxygen to form the more stable carbon dioxide (CO_2). Those who breathe too much carbon monoxide tend to die, fast or slow depending on the concentration. It strips oxygen molecules from the blood to form CO_2, which the body can't use and must exhale, at least until its oxygen runs out. The fact that the body considers CO_2 a waste product, by the way, doesn't say much for carbonated beverages.

Tap water is very low in oxygen, having no opportunity to be aerated during its journey through the pipes, and being loaded down with chlorine and various contaminants. Since cooking drives the extra oxygen out of vegetables, if one diet is mostly cooked or processed foods, there's yet another oxygen source lost.

Eating, Fasting and Oxygen Balance:

Overeating is so common in the US it's considered "normal". One cause is the widespread use of oral antibiotics. While destroying the target germs, these drugs also kill off one's intestinal flora, which are needed for healthy digestion. With these friendly bacteria gone, digestive efficiency plummets. As a result, the sensation of hunger comes more often and lasts longer, as the body tries to compensate for ineffective digestion by increasing the amounts consumed.

Even just eating daily, without ever giving the gastrointestinal tract a rest, loads down the blood with toxins and impurities, especially uric acid crystals. Under a microscope these resemble tiny coffin lids, interestingly enough, another clue to our Creator's whimsical sense of humor.

When the waste products exceed the cleansing capacity of the kidneys, the blood ends up just having to haul it around the body and stash it wherever possible. These toxins literally take up so much room in the blood cells that the cells can't take on enough oxygen when they pass through the lungs. The bloods primary function of picking up and distributing oxygen gets blocked by overuse of garbage-hauling function.

Fasting restores health by giving the overloaded blood cells a chance to dump the toxins and inert matter through normal organs of elimination at a rate they can handle, instead of through the skin, as in acne, or other inappropriate places. If the fast is long enough, accumulated residues in the body are also scoured out and expelled, giving a considerable spiritual resurgence once all the backlog is cleared away. While the debris is flushed out, various toxic reactions may come and go.

Once the blood is cleansed the red corpuscles have a lot more room for oxygen molecules, the oxygen saturation of the molecules is high, and health and energy are boosted considerably. Each breath now gives more life than it was able to in the blood's earlier state.

Most long-lived native peoples, who are not affected by our more common diseases, either include fasting as a regular part of their yearly food cycles, or eat much less overall, than industrialized peoples.

Today many Americans are existing at such high levels of toxicity, that their toxic reactions when attempting to fast can seem intense enough to make them start eating again before any serious cleansing can be accomplished.

243

Fortunately, one can partially bypass the lungs and get the blood level back up by taking oxygenated water internally and through the skin. Several weeks of detoxification by this regimen will also make it much easier to fast without discomfort, if one chooses. It reduces appetite, logically enough, to a level more in line with the body's actual needs. The bacteria that aid digestion are not killed by oral use of H2O2, as long as it's diluted properly.

Perhaps the greatest potential benefit (of H2O2 in water) is the reversal of the slight brain damage caused by long-term oxygen depletion, which can be observed in the "average" human, and is not always all that slight. It's well known that after about nine minutes of no oxygen, from drowning or whatever, you can kiss your brain good-bye. But the implications of constant gradual oxygen starvation in our cities somehow escape notice, despite the tiredness, depression, irritability, poor judgement and health problems affecting so many citizens.

Increasing the oxygen supply to the brain and nervous system will reverse these conditions. The oxywater regimen improves alertness, reflexes, memory and apparently intelligence, and may offer the elderly a new weapon against senility and related disorders. Alzheimer's and Parkinson's are reported to be responding to it. Alcoholics who start taking H2O2 soon lose interest in alcohol, and the thirst does not come back. Look up what alcohol does to your blood oxygen and your ability to use it, and you'll see why.

One possible spin-off of a coming major increase in the blood oxygen supply to human brains is that various short-sighted and oxygen-depleting activities such as deforestation, and other intelligent practices, should fade from the scene. Americans especially, will have an opportunity to outgrow many stupid things.

It's strange that the common drug aspirin "stops pain" by interfering with the nervous system's ability to use oxygen, in the electrochemical reactions needed to transmit impulses. Though maybe it's not that strange, considering that the Bayer Company which originated it was a subsidiary of IG Farben, the German chemical conglomerate that is famous for, among other things, developing and mass-producing the lethal gas Zyklon-B specifically for the exterminations at nazi death camps.

Economic Inertia: Dr. Terry McGrath, the CEO at Medizone, confirmed that hydrogen peroxide would in principle act much like ozone in destroying AIDS virus, but pointed out that it's never likely to be tested and proven in the laboratory. There's simply no economic incentive, since it's an unpatentable process and offers no more commercial returns than most other natural remedies. So it's completely up to individual patients and concerned citizens to push these options out into the open, immediately, before various companies get too financially committed to the assumption that AIDS (or any other disease) will continue to spread and be incurable. This is a good place as any for the FDA-required disclaimer: "Information given here is for research and educational purposes only and is not intended to prescribe treatment."

Veterinary And Agricultural Applications: Humans aren't the only life form to benefit from compensation for their oxygen deficient air, water and/or lifestyle. H2O2 in animals' drinking water, not enough to taste unpleasant, knocks out a growing list of illnesses. Locally, cats have gotten rid of their feline leukemia and chlamydia, and are back to their old energetic slapstick selves. Distemper in dogs has been reversed with H2O2, and a growing number of farmers are applying it to their livestock to cut losses from disease and infected wounds.

Plants grow better with an ounce of 3% H2O2 per quart of water they're given. Spray the solution on their leaves as well. Seeds germinate faster, with bigger sprouts, when they are first soaked in 1 ounce of 3% H2O2 to a pint of water. Instead of cutting trees that are diseased or otherwise struggling, spray them with H2O2 and water (1 part 3% to 32 parts water).

Why Isn't It Already In Use?: The obvious question is, if hyper-oxygenation is so simple and effective, why has it taken so long to discover it? Ozone is hardly new and hydrogen peroxide has been on the market for over a century. Why aren't all doctors already using it ? How come this story isn't all over the major news outlets?

Turning the question around helps clarify the problem. Just exactly what would happen if a cure was discovered that was completely effective against the vast majority of diseases, ridiculously cheap and plentiful, and in most cases could be self-administered without a physician? Would the current medical establishment welcome a breakthrough that could render 98% of all drugs, testing and disease related surgery obsolete? What would the response be of the pharmaceutical industrialists, hospital chain owners, health insurance moguls, AMA, and FDA?

Would you expect to read or hear such an announcement from any medical journal or media outlet owned by people financially committed to the medical status quo, which is practically all of them? How many want to make their own occupation unnecessary? And if the cure had already been suppressed once, wouldn't the possible blame for allowing people to die without it provide even more incentive to continue keeping the whole thing quiet?

All right then. This is precisely the situation that exists, and the cure has indeed been around for ages. It has been independently reported effective against virtually every disease at one time or another, in thousands of public-domain medical articles, which had never been collected or correlated until recently. And it is so simple and basic that concealing it from physicians and the general public has required a tremendous smoke screen of artificial complications, narrow specializations, symptomatic classifications and user hostile treatments.

If this is so, it follows that the more profit-fixed elements of the medical establishment will not be too thrilled about the recent surge in interest in oxygen therapies. The drug industry has expanded enormously since WWII, while America's level of health has dropped from the world's highest to the lowest among the industrialized nations. It does look as if the bottom line has been money and not health, for a long time.

The battle for the future of medicine, between Nature's truth and lucrative lies, is about to really heat up.

We can expect to see dis-information articles and news-casts with persuasive medical experts, some of whom will even believe what they're saying, warning of the dangers of hydrogen peroxide, ozone and even regular oxygen. These reports will attempt to blur the distinction between using therapeutic dosages at safe dilutions, and the harmful effects of excessive concentrations. Plenty of grisley examples are available, of what happens when various tissues are over-oxidized.

Anti-oxygenation propaganda pieces will probably not mention that over the years the FDA has approved H2O2 as a skin antiseptic at full 3% strength, as a hair bleaching agent at 6%, and for internal use as an additive for milk and in antiseptic long-shelf-life packaging. Nor are they likely to acknowledge that many European countries use ozone and H2O2 in their cities' water supply, and that they enjoy much better health than in the US. And they will be unable to truthfully cite any examples of people who were harmed by using H2O2 in the current demonstrated therapeutic concentrations.

If not enough of the public moves quickly to help spread the news of this alternative, those who fear that it could reduce their economic power may go so far as to try to knock off someone who promotes it, while trying to make it look like "too much oxygen" is the cause. Also, product tampering has thus far mostly targeted Bayer Aspirin's competitors, in case you hadn't noticed, but drug-store hydrogen peroxide would not be immune to such tactics.

One approach might be to plant a contaminated batch in a town where oral use is catching on and the medical establishment is losing ground, so someone gets hurt and the story gets nationwide coverage.

It is vital for Americans to realize that current economic dynamics don't allow the businessmen in charge of health and industry any incentive at all to make people permanently healthy and lose them as customers. It's the same reason why the energy conglomerates do not encourage citizens to become energy-self-sufficient, the Pentagon has no incentive to stop wars, and the American Psychiatric Association sees no advantage to ending mental illness.

Fortunately, the majority of physicians really do want to see their patients get well. They also wouldn't mind gaining the respect and admiration with which physicians were once widely regarded. When it comes down to choice between saving lives and protecting profits, most will be brave enough to overhaul their medical belief systems, discard obsolete methodologies, and basically tell the pharmaceutical conglomerates to go shove it. The rest will simply get left behind.

Further Information Sources:

1. "ECHO", a newsletter on Oxygen Therapy, is available from Walter Grotz, Box 126, Delano, MN 55328, (1$, 8p); 612-635-9297) have extensive references and case histories of successful treatments.

2. "The Peroxide Story" George L Borell, 3035 Rome Ave, Anaheim, CA 92804; 60 pp, $4.95 plus $1 postage.

3. The International Bio-Oxidative Medicine Foundation (IBOM) Newsletter contains technical updates for physicians using H2O2 therapies on their patients. PO Box 61767, Dallas/Ft. Worth, TX 75261; 817-481-9772.

4. Rex Research (PO Box 1258, Berkely, CA 94701) has five folios on Ozone Therapy; #4 ($2, 10 pp) is specifically on ozone treatment of AIDS; see also #1, ozone vs a wide variety of conditions (6$, 55pp); #2, ozone vs herpes, hepatitis, rheumatic diseases, also dental use ($4, 29pp); #3, cardiovascular, ozone enrichment of blood prior to transfusion (4$, 23 pp) and Ozone vs Cancer ($6, 55pp).

5. The International Ozone Association, 83 Oakwood Ave, Norwalk, CT 06850; (203-847-8169) has available "Medical Applications of Ozone" the largest single volume on the subject, for $50.

6. "Self-Treatment for AIDS: Oxygen Therapy" ($12.95, 100pp), and home remedies for Candida" ($8.95, 112pp) consist mostly of article reprints, compiled by Betsy Manning, 1600 Larkin #104, S.F. CA 94109.

7. "Search for Health", APW, PO Box 3052, Iowa City, Iowa 52244. Tom Valentine, Editor. Includes info on other oxygenating compounds for internal use, including AEROX, which they sell, and which is reported to give the same benefits as H2O2, but tastes better and is more stable, though more expensive. (We have not yet obtained a sample for testing.) APW also is a source for full-spectrum health-enhancing KIVA lights.

Some of the formal medical articles on H2O2 include:

"Hydrogen peroxide mediated killing of bacteria", D P Clifford and J E Repine, (Molecular and Cellular Biochemistry 49, 143-149, 1982)

"Generation of H2O2 in Biomembranes", T Ramasarma, (Biochemica et Biophysica Acta, 694, 1982, 69-93)

"Removal of Cholesterol and Other Lipids from Experimental Animal and Human Atheromatous Arteries by Dilute Hydrogen Peroxide", James W Finney, Bruce E Jay, et al, (Baylor University Medical Center, Dallas, Texas)

Also a series on the role of H2O2 in immunity to malaria, in The Lancet, 12/25/82 p 1431-1433, 1/29/83 p 234, and 2/12/83 p 359-360.

Medizone International, 123 East 54th St, Suite 2B, NY, NY 10022; 212-421-0303; issues shareholder reports updating the stateside verification of ozone blood treatment. Hansler ozone generators will also be available to licensed physicians through Medizone.

OXYGEN THERAPY UPDATE: Fall 1997

While assorted tentacles of the medical and media establishments are ineffectively thrashing around "looking for cures" for cancer, AIDS or whatever, countless thousands of people have gone ahead and eliminated their officially incurable conditions by sharply raising their internal oxidation rates. All disease-inducing microbes are unable to survive in fluids with high oxygen saturations, it turns out, while cells of higher life forms, and we'll presume that includes humans, all thrive at high oxygen levels.

In the nine years since "Hyper-Oxidation" was first printed and turned loose in Now What #1, considerable progress has been made with oxidative therapies. The main barriers to their broad adoption are the health industry's financial commitment to highly profitable conventional treatments, the insurance and advertising industries' resulting priorities, the institutionalized smothering of innovation and society's collective paralysis as mass belief systems gradually fall apart.

Oxygen therapies are quietly catching on in many areas now. A broad assortment of treatments involving ozone (O_3), hydrogen peroxide (H_2O_2) and other active oxygen supplements has gained innumerable enthusiasts, from informed citizens treating themselves to practitioners in virtually all medical specialties. However, the majority of these tend to maintain low profiles to avoid tangling with enforcers of medical conventionality. So for now, any lists of physicians offering oxygen therapies are limited to those willing to take on whatever risks go with being on such lists. Nevertheless, growing numbers of health care providers are utilizing these unapproved but most effective methods.

Several states have overridden the FDA's prohibition on ozone therapy and its use is spreading among physicians who are grasping the liberating implications of why we breathe oxygen. One highly effective connection among these is Dr. John C. Pittman who heads an association of physicians and patients who joined forces to help publicize oxidative therapies and remove legal barriers to their wider implementation. Dr. Pittman is at 4504 Fair Meadow Lane, Suite 111, Raleigh, NC 17607; (919) 571-4391.

The growing public awareness of and enthusiasm for H2O2 is apparently starting to wear down the FDA's resistance; they (FDA) have begun certifying doctors for delivery of H2O2 IV's (250 cc of 0.035% H2O2 infused over a half an hour.) An H2O2 IV has been described as accomplishing the same effect as two weeks of the oral regimen. As with other oxidative therapies, the results are not so much due to the amount of oxygen administered, but to the catalytic effect of electrically active oxygen raising the body's own oxidative processes closer to the range where health prevails. Physicians offering H2O2 IV's may be contacted through the International Bio-Oxidative Medicine Foundation (IBOM) at P.O. Box 13205, Oklahoma City, OK 73113-1205; (405) 478-4266.

However, despite efforts to get the mass media onto this story, as far as the media is concerned, oxygen therapies do not exist and there's still no cure for cancer, AIDS, alzheimer's, etc. Those who profit by perpetuating wide public belief that many diseases are inherently incurable have outspent by literally a million to one those of us trying to spread the truth that there really is a cure, it just happens to be unpatentable, unprofitable and right under everyone's nose.

Thus, the people whose news sources are limited to the mass media and who aren't lucky enough to hear about ozone and H2O2 through some other channel, are out there still suffering and dying needlessly. What's spent on a year's advertisements for cold remedies alone would eliminate colds altogether, along with quite a few other disorders, if invested in oxygen therapies. One hundredth the ink or air time spent on the "assisted suicide" issue, (as if that were the only alternative,) could have saved millions of lives and billions of pain-hours if spent instead on showing how therapies using oxygen have cured people of the very things patients have sought suicide to escape from.

Waves Forest
Fall, 1997

For more information on oxygen therapies check out the following sources:

"Hydrogen Peroxide: Medical Miracle" by William Campbell Douglas, M.D. available from Second Opinion Publishing, Suite 100, 1350 Center Drive, Dunwoods, GA 30338.

"The Use of Ozone in Medicine" by Dr. Siegfreid Rilling, M.D., Ph.D. and Renate Viebahn, Ph.D. from Haug Publishers, the English Version from Medicina Biologica, 2937 N.E. Flanders Street, Portland, OR 97232.

Appendix VI:

Dr. Otto Warburg, Ph.D.
"On the Origin of Cancer Cells,"

SCIENCE
(February 4, 1956)
Volume 13, Number 3191,
pp. 309-314.

Professor Otto Warburg was the director of the Max Planck Institute for Cell Physiology, Berlin-Dahlem, Germany. This article is based on a lecture delivered at Stuttgart on May 25, 1955, before the German Central Committee for Cancer Control. It was first published in German [Naturwissenschaften 42, 401 (1955)]. This translation was prepared by Dean Burk, Jehu Hunter, and W.Wh. Everhardy of the United States Department of Health, Education, and Welfare, Public Health Service, National Institutes of Health, Bethesda, Maryland, with permission of Naturwissenschaften and with collaboration of Professor Warburg, who introduced additional material.

Our principal experimental object for the measurement of the metabolism of cancer cells is today no longer the tumor, but the ascites cancer cells (1) living free in the abdominal cavity, which are almost pure cultures of cancer cells with which one can work quantitatively as in chemical analysis. Formerly it could be said of tumors, with their varying cancer cell content, that they ferment more strongly the more cancer cells they contain, but today we can determine the absolute fermentation values of the cancer cells and find such high values that we come very close to the fermentation values of wildly proliferating Torula yeasts.

What was formerly only qualitative has now become quantitative. What was formerly only probable has now become certain. The era in which the fermentation of the cancer cells or its importance could be disputed is over, and no one today can doubt that we understand the origin of cancer cells if we know how their large fermentation originates, or, to express it more fully, if we know how the damaged respiration and the excessive fermentation of the cancer cells originate.

Energy of Respiration and Fermentation: We now understand the chemical mechanisms of respiration and fermentation almost completely, but we do not need this knowledge for what follows, since energy alone will be the center of our consideration. We need to know no more of respiration and fermentation here than that they are energy-producing reactions and that they synthesize the energy-rich adenosine triphosphate (A.T.P.), through which the energy of respiration and fermentation is then made available for life.

Since it is known how much adenosine triphosphate can be synthesized by respiration and how much by fermentation, we can write immediately the potential, biologically utilizable energy production of any cells if we have measure their respiration and fermentation rates. With the ascites cancer cells of the mouse, for example, we find an average respiration rate of seven cubic millimeters of oxygen consumed per milligram, per hour, and a fermentation rate of 60 cubic millimeters of lactic acid produced per milligram, per hour. This, converted to energy equivalents, means that the cancer cells can obtain approximately the same amount of energy from fermentation as from respiration, whereas the normal body cells obtain much more energy from respiration than from fermentation. For example, the liver and the kidney of an adult animal obtain about 100 times as much energy from respiration as from fermentation.

I shall not consider aerobic fermentation, which is a result of the interaction of respiration and fermentation, because aerobic fermentation is too labile and too dependent on external conditions. Of importance for the considerations that follow are only the two stable independent metabolic processes, respiration and anaerobic fermentation: respiration, which is measured by the oxygen consumption of cells that are saturated with oxygen; and fermentation, which is measured by the formation of lactic acid in the absence of oxygen.

Injuring of Respiration: Since the respiration of all cancer cells is damaged, our firm question is, "How can the respiration of body cells be injured?" Of this damage to respiration, it can be said at the outset that it must be irreversible, since the respiration of cancer cells can never return to normal.

Second, the injury to respiration must not be so great that the cells are killed, for then no cancer cells could result. If respiration is damaged when it forms too little adenosine triphosphate, it may be either that the oxygen consumption has been decreased or that, with undiminished oxygen consumption, the coupling between respiration and the formation of adenosine triphosphate has been broken, as was first pointed out by Feodor Lynen (2).

One method for the destruction of the respiration of body cells is removal of oxygen. If, for example, embryonal tissue is exposed to an oxygen deficiency for some hours, and then is placed in oxygen again, 50 percent more of the respiration is destroyed.

The cause of this destruction of respiration is lack of energy. As a matter of fact, the cells need their respiratory energy to preserve their structure, and if respiration is inhibited, both structure and respiration disappear.

Another method for destroying respiration is to use respiratory poisons. From the standpoint of energy, this method comes to the same result as the first method. No matter whether oxygen is withdrawn from the cell or whether the oxygen is prevented from reacting by a poison, the result is the same in both cases-namely, impairment of respiration from lack of energy.

I may mention a few respiratory poisons. A strong, specific respiratory poison is arsenious acid, which as every clinician knows, may produce cancer. Hydrogen sulfide and many of its derivatives are also strong, specific respiratory poisons. We know today that certain hydrogen sulfide derivatives, thiourea and thioacetamide, with which citrus fruit juices have been preserved in recent times, induce cancer of the liver and gall bladder in rats.

Urethane is a nonspecific respiratory poison. It inhibits respiration as a chemically indifferent narcotic, since it displaces metabolites from cell structures. In recent years, it has been recognized that subnarcotic doses of urethane

258

cause lung cancer in mice in 100 percent of treatments. Urethane is particularly suitable as a carcinogen, because in contrast to alcohol, it is not itself burned up on the respiring surfaces , and, unlike ether or chloroform, it does not cytolize the cells. Any narcotic that has these properties may cause cancer upon chronic administration in small doses.

The first notable experimental induction of cancer by oxygen deficiency was described by Goldblatt and Cameron (3), who exposed heart fibroblasts in tissue culture to intermittent oxygen deficiency for long periods, and finally obtained transplantable cancer cells, whereas in control cultures that were maintained without oxygen deficiency, no cancer cells resulted. Clinical experiences along these lines are innumerable: the production of cancer by intermittent irritation of the outer skin and of the mucosa of internal organs, by the plugging of the excretory ducts of glands, by cirrhoses of tissues, and so forth. In all these cases, the intermittent irritation lead to intermittent circulatory disturbances. Probably chronic intermittent oxygen deficiency plays a greater role in the formation of cancer in the body than does the chronic administration of respiratory poisons.

Any respiratory injury due to lack of energy, however, whether it is produced by oxygen deficiency or by respiratory poisons, must be cumulative, since it is irreversible. Frequent, small doses of respiratory poisons are therefore more dangerous than a single large dose, where there is always the chance that the cells will be killed rather than that they will become carcinogenic.

Grana: If an injury of respiration is to produce cancer, this injury must, as already mention, be irreversible. We understand by this not only that the inhibition of respiration remains after removal of the respiratory poison, but, even more, that the inhibition of respiration also continues through all the following cell division, for measurements of metabolism in transplanted tumors have shown that cancer cells cannot regain normal respiration, even in the course of many decades, once they have lost it.

This originally mysterious phenomenon has been explained by a discovery that comes from the early years of cell physiology (4). When liver cells were cytolized by infusion of water and the cytolyzate was centrifuged, it was found that the greater part of the respiration sank to the bottom with the cell grana.

It was also shown that the respiration of the centrifuged grana was inhibited by narcotics at concentrations affecting cell structures, from which it was concluded - already in 1914- that the respiring grana are not insoluble cell particles but autonomous organisms, a result that has been extended in recent years by the English botanist Darlington (5) and particularly by Mark Woods and H.G. du Buy (6) of the National Cancer Institute in Bethesda, Maryland.

Woods and du Buy have experimentally expanded our concepts concerning the self-perpetuating nature of mitochondrial elements (grana) and have demonstrated the hereditary role of extranuclear aberrant forms of these in the causation of neoplasia. The autonomy of the respiring grana, both biochemically and genetically, can hardly be doubted today.

If the principle "Omne granum e grano" is valid for respiring grana, we understand why the respiration connected with grana remains damaged when it has once been damaged; it is for the same reason that properties linked with genes remain damaged when the genes have been damaged.

Furthermore, the connection of respiration with the grana (7) also explains carcinogenesis that I have not mentioned previously, the carcinogenesis is causedby x-rays. Rajewsky and Pauly have recently shown that the respiration linked with the grana can be destroyed with strong doses of x-rrays, while the small part of the respiration that takes place in the fluid protoplasm can be inhibited very little by irradiation. Carcinogenesis by X-rays is obviously nothing else than destruction of respiration by elimination of the respiring grana.

It should also be mentioned here that grana, as Graffi has shown (8), fluoresce brightly if carcinogenic hydrocarbons are brought into their surroundings, because the grana accumulate the carcinogenic substances. Probably this accumulation is the explanation for the fact that carcinogenic hydrocarbons, although almost insoluble in water, can inhibit respiration and therefore have a carcinogenic effect.

Increase of Fermentation: When the respiration of body cells has been irreversibly damaged, cancer cells by no means immediately result. For cancer formation, there is necessary not only an irreversible damaging of the respiration, but also an increase in the fermentation -- indeed, such an increase of the fermentation that the failure of respiration is compensated for energetically. But how does this increase of fermentation come about?

The most important fact in this field is that there is no physical or chemical agent with which the fermentation of cells in the body can be increased directly; for increasing fermentation, a long time and many cell divisions are always necessary. The temporal course of this increase of fermentation in carcinogenesis has been measured in many interesting works, among which I should like to make special mention of those of Dean Burk (9). Burk first cut out part of the liver of healthy rats and investigated the metabolism of the liver cells in the course of ensuing regeneration, in which, as is well known, the liver grows more rapidly than a rapidly growing tumor.

No increase of fermentation was found. Burk then fed rats for 200 days on yellow butter, whereupon liver carcinomas were produced, and he found that the fermentation slowly increased in the course of 200 days toward values characteristic of tumors.

The mysterious latency period of the production of cancer is, therefore, nothing more than the time in which the fermentation increases after a damaging of the respiration. This time differs in various animals: it is essentially long in man and here often amounts to several decades, as can be determined by the cases in which the time of the respiratory damage is known - for example, in arsenic cancer and irradiation cancer.

The driving force of the increase of fermentation, however, is the energy deficiency under which the cells operate after destruction of their respiration which forces the cells to replace the irretrievably lost respiration energy in some way. They are able to do this by a selective process that makes use of the fermentation of the normal body cells.

The more weakly fermenting body cells perish, but the more strongly fermenting ones remain alive, and this selective process continues until respiratory failure is compensated for energetically by the increase in fermentation. Only then has a cancer cell resulted from the normal body cell.

Now we understand why the increase in fermentation takes such a long time and why it is possible only with the help of many cell divisions. We also understand why the latency period is different in rats and in man. Since the average fermentation of normal rat cells is much greater than the average fermentation of normal human cells, the selective process begins at a higher fermentation level in the rat and, hence is completed more quickly than it is in man.

It follows from this that there would be no cancers if there were no fermentation of normal body cells, and hence we should like to know, naturally, from where the fermentation of the normal body cells stems and what its significance is in the body. Since, as Burk has shown, the fermentation remains almost zero in the regenerating liver growth, we must conclude that the fermentation of the body cells is greatest in the very earliest stages of embryonal development. Under these conditions, it is obvious -- since ontogeny is the repetition of phylogeny-- that the fermentation of body cells is the inheritance of undifferentiated ancestors that have lived in the past at the expense of fermentation energy.

Structure and Energy: But why -- and this is our last question -- are the body cells differentiated when their respiration energy is replaced by fermentation energy?

At first, one would think that it is immaterial to the cells whether they obtain their energy from respiration in or from fermentation, since the energy of both reactions is transformed into the energy of adenosine triphosphate, and yet adenosine triphosphate = adenosine triphosphate. This equation is certainly correct chemically and energetically, but it is incorrect morphologically, because although respiration takes place for the most part in the structure of the grana, the fermentation enzymes are found for a greater part in the fluid protoplasm.

The adenosine triphosphate is synthesized by fermentation. Thus, it is as if one reduced the same amount of silver on a photographic plate by the same amount of light, but in one case with diffused light and in the other with patterned light.

In the first case, a diffuse blackening appears on the plate, but in the second case, a picture appears; however, the same thing happens chemically and energetically in both cases. Just as one type of light energy involves more structure than the other type, the adenosine triphosphate energy involves more structure when it is formed by respiration than it does when it is formed by fermentation.

In any event, it is one of the fundamental facts of present-day biochemistry that adenosine triphosphate can be synthesized in homogeneous solutions with crystallized fermentation enzymes, whereas so far no one has succeeded in synthesizing adenosine triphosphate in homogeneous solutions with dissolved respiratory enzymes, and the structure always goes with oxidative phosphorylation.

Moreover, it was known for a long time before the advent of crystallized fermentation enzymes and oxidative phosphorylation that fermentation --the energy supplying reaction of the lower organisms -- is morphologically inferior to respiration. Not even yeast, which is one of the lowest forms of life, can maintain its structure permanently by fermentation alone; it degenerates to bizarre forms.

However, as Pasteur showed, it is rejuvenated in a wonderful manner, if it comes in contact with oxygen for a short time. "I should not be surprised," Pasteur said in 1886 (10) in the description of these experiments, "if there should arise in the mind of an attentive hearer a presentiment about the causes of those great mysteries of life which we conceal under the words youth and age of cells." Today, after 80 years, the explanation is as follows: the firmer connection of respiration with structure and the looser connection of fermentation with structure.

This, therefore, is the physiochemical explanation of the dedifferentiation of cancer cells. If the structure of yeast cannot be maintained by fermentation alone, one need not state that highly differentiated body cells lose their differentiation upon continuous replacement of their respiration with fermentation.

I would like at this point to draw attention to a consequence of practical importance. When one irradiates a tissue that contains cancer cells as well as normal cells, the respiration of the cancer cells, already too small, will decline further. If the respiration falls below a certain minimum that the cells need unconditionally, despite their increased fermentation, they die; whereas the normal cells, where respiration may be harmed by the same amount, will survive because, with a greater initial respiration, they will still possess a higher residual respiration after irradiation. This explains the selective killing action of x-rays on cancer cells. But still further: the descendants of the surviving normal cells may in the course of the latent period compensate the respiration decrease by the fermentation increase and, thence, become cancer cells.

Thus it happens that radiation, which kills cancer cells, can also at the same time produce cancer, or that urethane, which kills cancer cells, can also at the same time produce cancer. Both events take place from harming respiration: the killing, by harming an already harmed respiration; the carcinogenesis, by the harming of a not yet harmed respiration.

Maintenance Energy: When differentiation of the body cells has occurred and cancer cells have thereby developed, there appears a phenomenon to which our attention has been called by the special living conditions of ascites cancer cells. In extensively progressed ascites cancer cells of the mouse, the abdominal cavity contains so many cancer cells that the latter cannot utilize their full capacity to respire, and ferment because of the lack of oxygen and sugar. Nevertheless, the cancer cells remain alive in the abdominal cavity, as the result of transplantation proves.

Recently, we have confirmed this result by direct experiments in which we placed varying amounts of energy at the disposal of the ascites outside the body, in vitro, and then transplanted it. This investigation showed that all cancer cells were killed when no energy at all was supplied for 24 hours at 38 degrees Celsius but that one-fifth of the growth energy was sufficient to preserve the transplantability of the ascites.

This result can also be expressed by saying that cancer cells require much less energy to keep them alive than they do for growth. In this they resemble other lower cells, such as yeast cells, which remain alive for a long time in densely packed packets -- almost without respiration and fermentation.

In any case, the ability of cancer cells to survive with little energy, if they are not growing, will be of great importance for the behavior of the cancer cells in the body.

Sleeping Cancer Cells: Since the increase in fermentation in the development of cancer cells takes place gradually, there must be a transitional phase between normal body cells and fully formed cancer cells. Thus, for example, when fermentation has become so great that the respiration defect has been fully compensated for energetically by fermentation, we may have cells which indeed look like cancer cells but are still energetically insufficient. Such cells, which are clinically not cancer cells, have lately been found, not only in the prostate, but also in the lungs, kidney, and stomach of elderly persons. Such cells have been referred to as "sleeping cancer cells." (11, 12)

The sleeping cancer cells will possibly play a role in chemotherapy. From energy consideration, I could think that sleeping cancer cells could be killed more easily than growing cancer cells in the body, and that the most suitable test objects for finding effective agents would be the sleeping cells of the skin -- that is, the precancerous skin.

Summary: Cancer cells originate from normal body cells in two phases. The first phase is the irreversible injuring of respiration. Just as there are many remote causes of plague --heat, insects, rats-- but only one common cause, the plague bacillus, there are a great many remote causes of cancer --tar, x-rays, arsenic, pressure, urethane-- but there is only one common cause into which all other causes of cancer merge, the irreversible injuring of respiration.

The irreversible injuring of respiration is followed, as the second phase of cancer formation, by a long struggle for existence by the injured cells to maintain their structure, in which a part of the cells perish from lack of energy, while another part succeed in replacing the irretrievably lost respiration by fermentation energy. Because of the morphological inferiority of fermentation energy, the highly differentiated body cells are converted by this into undifferentiated cells that grow wildly -- the cancer cells.

To the thousands of quantitative experiments on which these results are based, I should like to add, as a further argument, the fact that there is no alternative today. If the explanation of a vital process is its reduction to physics and chemistry, there is today no other explanation for the origin of cancer cells, either special or general. From this point of view, mutation and carcinogenic agent are not alternatives, but empty words, unless metabolically specified. Even more harmful in the struggle against cancer can be the continual discovery of miscellaneous cancer agents and cancer viruses, which, by obscuring the underlying phenomena, may hinder necessary preventive measures and thereby become responsible for cancer cases.

Technical Considerations And Comments

Metabolism of the ascites cancer cells: The high fermentation of ascites cancer cells was discovered in Dahlem in 1951 (12) and since then has been confirmed in many works (13,14). For best measurements, the ascites cells are not transferred to Ringer's solution but are maintained in their natural medium, ascites serum, which is adjusted physiologically at the beginning of the measurement by addition of glucose and bicarbonate. Because of the very large fermentation, it is necessary to dilute the ascites cells that are removed from the abdominal cavity rather considerably with ascites serum; otherwise the bicarbonate would be used up within a few minutes after addition to the glucose, and hence the fermentation would be brought to a standstill.

Under physiological conditions of pH and temperature, we find the following metabolic quotients in ascites serum (15):

$$QQ(O2) = -5 \text{ to } -10$$
$$Q(M)(O2) = 25 \text{ to } 35$$
$$Q(M)(N2) = 50 \text{ to } 70$$

where $Q(O2)$ is the amount of oxygen in cubic millimeters that 1 milligram of tissues (dry weight) consumes per hour at 38 degrees Celsius with oxygen saturation, $Q(M)(O2)$ is the amount of lactic acid in cubic millimeters that 1 milligram of tissue (dry weight) develops per hour at 38 degrees Celsius in the absence of oxygen. Even higher fermentation quotients have been found in the United States with other strains of mouse ascites cancer cells (13,14).

All calculations of the energy-production potential of cancer cells should now be based on quotients of the ascites cancer cells, since these quotients are 2 or 3 times as large anaerobically as the values formerly found for the purest solid tumors. The quotients of the normal body cells, however, remain as they were found in Dahlem in the years from 1924 to 1929 (16-19). It is clear that the difference in metabolism between normal cells and cancer cells is much greater than it formerly appeared to be on the basis of measurements of solid tumors.

Utilizable energy of respiration and fermentation: Since the discovery of the oxidation reaction of fermentation in 1939 (20), we have known the chemical reactions by which adenosine diphosphate (A.D.P.) is phosphorylated to adenosine triphosphate in fermentation; and since then we have found that 1 mole of fermentation lactic acid produces 1 mole of adenosine triphosphate (A.T.P.).

The chemical reactions by which A.T.P. is synthesized in respiration are still unknown, but it can be assumed, according to the existing measurements (21), that 7 moles of A.T.P. can be formed when 1 mole of oxygen is consumed in respiration.

A.T.P. quotients: If we multiply Q(O2) by 7 and Q(M)(N2) by 1, we obtain the number of cubic millimeters of A.T.P. that 1 milligram of tissue (dry substance) can synthesize per hour (22,400 cubic millimeters=1 millimole of A.T.P.). We call these quotients Q(A.T.P.) (O2) and Q(A.T.P.)(N2), according to whether the A.T.P. is formed by respiration or by fermentation, respectively.

Energy production of cancer cells and normal body cells: In Table 1, the Q values of some normal body cells are contrasted with the Q values of our ascites cancer cells.

The cancer cells have about as much energy available as the normal body cells, but the ratio of the fermentation energy to the respiration energy is much greater in the cancer cells than it is in the normal cells.

Uncoupling of respiration: If a young rat embryo is transferred from the amniotic sac to Ringer's solution, the previously transparent embryo becomes opaque and soon appears coagulated (17). At the same time, the connection between respiration and phosphorylation is broken; that is, although oxygen is still consumed and carbon dioxide is still developed, the energy of this combustion process is lost for life. If the metabolism quotients had previously been in the amniotic fluid:

$Q(O2) = -15, Q(M)(O2) = 25, Q(M)(N2) = 25$
$Q(A.T.P.)(O2) = 105, Q(A.T.P.)(N2) = 25$

afterward in Ringer's solution they are:

$Q(O2) = -15, Q(M)(O2) = 25, Q(M)(N2) = 25$
$Q(A.T.P.)(O2) = 0, Q(A.T.P.)(N2) = 25$

Because of uncoupling of respiration and phosphorylation, the energy production of the embryo has fallen from $Q(ZA.T.P.)(O2) = Q(A.T.P.)(N2) = 130$, to 51; since the uncoupling is irreversible, the embryo dies in the Ringer's solution.

This example will show that the first phase of carcino-genesis, the irreversible damaging of respiration, need not be an actual decrease in the respiration quotient but merely an uncoupling of respiration, with undiminished overall oxygen consumption. Ascites cancer cells, which owe their origin primarily to an uncoupling of respiration, could conceivably have the following metabolism quotients, for example:

$$Q(O2) = -50, Q(M)(O2) = 100, Q(M)(N2) = 100$$
$$Q(A.T.P.)(O2), Q(A.T.P.)(N2) = 100$$

which would mean that, despite great respiration, the usable energy production would be displaced completely toward the side of fermentation. One will now have to search for such cancer cells among the ascites cancer cells. Solid tumors -- and especially solid spontaneous tumors-- need no longer be subjected to such examinations today, of course, since the solid tumors are usually so impure histologically.

Aerobic fermentation: Aerobic fermentation is a property of all growing cancer cells, but aerobic fermentation [p.313 -->] without growth is a property of damaged body cells -- for example, embryos that have been transferred from amniotic fluid to Ringer's solution.

Since it is always easy to detect aerobic fermentation but generally difficult to detect growth, or lack thereof, of body cells, aerobic fermentation should not be used as a test for cancer cells, as I made clear in 1928 (19).

Nevertheless, misuse is still made of aerobic fermentation. Thus, O'Connor (22) recently repeated our old experiments on the aerobic fermentation of the embryo that has been transferred into Ringer's solution, but he drew the conclusion that the growth of normal body cells is completed at the expense of the aerobic fermentation, even though it has long been established that the embryo does not ferment aerobically when it grows in the amniotic fluid.

Oxygen deficiency: Short-period oxygen deficiency irreversibly destroys the respiration of embryos (16) without thereby inhibiting the anaerobic fermentation of the embryo. If such embryos are transplanted, teratomas are formed (31). It has recently been reported that, in the development of the Alpine salamander, malformations occurred when the respiration was inhibited by hydrocyanic acid in the early stages of embryonal development (32).

Goldblatt and Cameron (3) reported that, in the in vitro culturing of fibroblasts, tumor cells appeared when the cultures were exposed to intermittent oxygen deficiency for long periods, whereas, in the control cultures, no tumor cells appeared. In the discussion at the Stuttgart convention, Lettre cited against Goldblatt and Cameron the fact that another American tissue culturist, Earle, had occasionally obtained tumor cells from fibroblasts for reasons unknown to him and in an unreproduceable manner, but this objection does not seem weighty, and the latter part is untrue (33). In any event, here is an area in which the methods of tissue culture could prove useful for cancer research. But warnings must be given against metabolism measurements in tissue cultures, if and when the tissue cultures are mixtures of growing and dying cells, especially under conditions of malnutrition. An example of the latter type of confusion is involved in the discussion by Albert Fischer (34), especially in the chapter "Energy exchange of tissue cells cultivated in vitro."

Addendum in vitro carcinogenesis and metabolism: Since this paper was prepared, striking confirmation and extension of its main conclusions have been obtained from correlated metabolic and growth studies of two lines of tissue culture cancer cells of widely differing malignancy that were both derived from one and the same normal, tissue culture cell (36). The single cell as isolated some 5 years ago from a 97-day old parent culture of a strain C3H/He mouse by Sanford, Likkely and Earle (33) of the National Cancer Institute.

Up to the time that the single-cell isolation was made, no tumors developed when cells of the parent culture were injected into strain C3H/He mice. Injections of in vitro cells of the lines 1742 and 049 (formerly labeled substrains VII and III, respectively) first produced tumors in normal C3H/He mice after the 12th and 19th in vitro transplant generations, respectively after 1.5 years, the percentage production of sarcomas was 63 and 0 percent, respectively, with correspondingly marked differences in length of induction period.

Despite such gross differences in "malignancy" in vivo, the rates of growth of the two lines of cells maintained continuously in vitro have remained nearly identical and relatively rapid. Nevertheless, the metabolism of the two lines of cancer cells, whose malignancy was developed in vitro, has been found by Woods, Hunter, Hobby, and Burk to parallel strikingly the differences in malignancy observed in vivo, in a manner in harmony with the predications and predictions of this article.

The metabolic values were measured following direct transfer of the liquid cultures from the growth flasks into manometric vessels, without notable alteration of environmental temperature, pH, or medium composition (horse serum, chick embryo extract, glucose, bicarbonate, balanced saline). The values obtained this way accurately represent the metabolism of growing, adequately nourished, pure lines of healthy cancer cells free of admixture with any other tissue cell type. The anaerobic glycolysis of the high-malignancy line 1742 was $Q(M)N2 = 60$ to 80, which is virtually maximum for any and all cancer cells previously reported, including ascites cells (12-14). The anaerobic glycolysis of the low -malignancy line was, however, only one-third as great, $Q(M)N2 = 20$ to 30. The average aerobic glycolysis values for the two lines were in the the same order, $Q(M)O2 = 30$ and 10, respectively, but of lower magnitude because of the usual, pronounced Pasteur effect, greater in line 1742 than in line 2049 [$Q(M)N2 - Q(M)O2 = $ about 40 and 15]. On the other hand, the rates of oxygen consumption were in converse order, being smaller in line 1742 [$Q(O2) = 5$ to 10] than in line 2049 [$Q(O2) = 10$ to 15], corresponding to a greater degree of respiratory defect in line 1742.

The respiratory defect in both lines was further delineated by the findings of little or no increase in respiration after the addition of succinate to either line of cells, in contrast to the considerable increases obtained with virtually all normal tissues (9); and the respiratory increase with paraphenylenediamine was likewise relatively low, compared with normal tissue responses.

A further notable difference between the two cell lines was the very much lower inhibition of glycolysis by podophyllin materials (anti-insulin potentiators) observed with line 1742 compared with line 2049 (for example, 10 and 70 percent, respectively, at a suitably low concentration). This result would be expected on the basis of the much greater loss of anti-insulin hormonal restraint of glucose metabolism, at the hexokinase phosphorylating level, as the degree of malignancy is increased, just as was reported for a spectrum of solid tumors (14).

Finally, the high-malignancy line 1742 cells have been found by A. L. Schade to contain 3 times as much aldolase as the low-malignancy line 2049 cells (11,300 versus 3700 Warburg activity units per millimeter of packed cells extracted), and about 2 times as much a-glycerophosphate dehydrogenase [600 versus 1400 Schade activity units (13) per millimeter of packed cells extracted]. The potential significance of these indicated enzymic differences in relation to the parallel glycolytic differences, measured with aliquots of the same cell cultures, is evident, and may well be connected with the corresponding hexokinase system differences.

The new metabolic data on the two remarkably contrasting lines of cancer cells, which originated from a single, individual cell and have been maintained exclusively in vitro over a period of years, epitomize and prove finally the main conclusions of this article, which are based on decades of research. Such metabolic analyses provide promise of a powerful tool for diagnosis of malignancy in the ever-increasing variety of tissue culture lines now becoming available in this rapidly expanding biological and medical field, where characterization of malignancy by conventional methods (animal inoculation or otherwise) may be difficult or impracticable. This metabolic tool should be especially important in connection with the use of tissue cultures for the evaluation of chemotherapeutic agents or other control procedures.

References and Notes

1. The tranplantable ascites cancer was discovered by H. Loewenthal and G. Jahn [Z. Krebsforsch, 37,439 (1932)]. G. Klein (Stockholm) expanded our knowledge about the physiology and morphology of the ascites tumors and showed their great advantages as experimental material. [Exptl. Cell Research, 2, 518 (1951)]

2. F. Lynen, Naturwissenschaften 30, 398 (1942); Ann. Chem. Justus Liebig 573, 60 (1951).

3. H. Goldblatt and G. Cameron, J. Exptl. Med, 97, 525 (1953).

4. O. Warburg, Pfluger's. Arch. Ges. Physiolo. 154,599 (1913); 158, 19 (1914).

5. C.D. Darlington, Brit. J. Cancer 2, 118 (1948).

6. M.W. Woods et al., J. Natl. Cancer Inst., 11, 1105 (1951); 9, 311 (19949); 9, 325 (1949); 16, 351 (1955). Science 102, 591 (1945); 111, 572 (1950). AAAS Research Conf. On Cancer (Science Press, Lancaster, Pa., 19945), p. 162. J.

WASH. ACAD. SCI. 42, 169 (195). Pigment Cell Growth, M. Gordon, Ed. (Academic Press, New York, 1953), p.335. Biochem. Et Biophys. Acta 12, 329 (1953). Proc. Am. Ass. Cancer Research 1, 7 (1954). Proc. Soc. Exptl. Biol. Med. 83, 6 (1953). Phytopathology 33, 637, 766 (1943); 36, 47 (1946); 31, 978 (1941); 3, 288 (1942). Am. J. Botany 33, 12a (1946); 38, 419 (1951).

7.   A compilation of American works on the grana, in which my results of 1914 (4) have been confirmed, is given by G. Hogeboom, W. Schneider, and M. Striebich in Cancer Research [133, 617 (1953)]. In a very special case -- nucleated red blood cells of birds, which contain no grana or only poorly visible ones -- the entire respiration can be centrifuged off with the cell nuclei [O. Warburg, Hoppeseyler's Z. Physiol. Chem. 70, 413 (1913)].

8.   A. Graffi, Z. Krebsforsch, 49, 477 (1939).

9.   D. Burk, Symposium On Respiratory Enzymes (University of Wisconsin Press, Madison, 194), p.335. J. G. Kidd, R. J. Winzler, D. Burk, Cancer Research 4, 547 (1944).

10.   L. Pasteur, Etudes Sur La Bierre (Masson, Paris, 1876), p. 240.

11.   J. Craigie, J. Pathol. Bacteriol. 63, 177 (1951); 64, 251 (1952). H. Hamperl, Verhandl. Deut. Ges. Pathol. 35, 9 (1951).

12.   O. Warburg And E. Hiepler, Z. Naturforsch 7b, 193 (1952).

13.   A.l. Shade, Biochim. Et. Biophys. Acta 12, 163 (1953).

14.   M. Woods, J. Hunter, D. Burk, J. Natl. Cancer. Inst. 16, 351 (1955).

15. I am indebted to Georg Klein of the Karolinsska Instittute, Stockholm Sweden, for his Ehrlich strain of mouse ascites cells.

16. O, Warburg, K. Posener, E. Negelein, Biochem. Z. 152, 309 (1924).

17. E. Negelein, Ibid, 165, 122 (1925).

18. O. Warburg et al., Ibid, 189, 114, 175, 242 (1924); 193, 315 (1928); 197, 175 (1928); 204, 475, 479 (199).

19. O. Warburg, Ibid. 204, 482 (1929).

20. O. Warburg et al., Ibid. 303, 40, 132 (1939).

21. H.A. Krebs et al., Biochem. H. London 54, 107 (19953).

22. R.j. O'connor, Brit. J. Exptl.pathol. 31, 390 (1951).

23. O. Warburg, Hoppe-seyler's Z. Physiol. Chem. 70, 413 (1911); M. Onaka, Ibid. 70, 433 (1911); 71, 1933 (1911).

24. K. Dresel, Biochem. Z. 178, 70 (1926).

25. E. Negelein, Ibid. 165, 203 (1925).

26. D.N. Gupta, Nature 175, 257 (1955)..

27. R. Usui, Pfluger's Arch. Ges. Physiol. 147, 100 (1912).

28. O. Warburg, Hoppe-steyler's Z. Physiol. Chem. 66, 305 (1910); 70, 413 (1911).

29. ----------, Biochem. 119, 143 (1921).

30. C.D. Larsen, J. Natl. Cancer Inst. 8, 63 (1947).

31. O. Warburg, Biochem. Z. 2288, 257 (1930).

32. H. Tiedemann And H. Tiedemann, Z. Natursforsch. 9b, 371 (1954).

33. K.k. Sanford, G.d. Likely, W.R. Earle, J. Natl. Cancer Inst. 15, 15 (1954).

34. A. Fischer, Biology Of Tissue Culture (Copenhagen, Denmark, 1946).

35. O. Warburg, Biochem. Z. 160, 307 (1925); D. Burk et al., J. Natl. Cancer Inst. 2, 201 (1941).

36. This summary of studies of various collaborative groups of investigators was prepared by Dean Burk at Professor Warburg's request.

Please Note: The author does not intentionally state nor infer in any way that oxygen-based therapies and/or oxygen supplementation will control, reduce or cure cancer. This article, by Dr. Warburg, is included in this book to clarify the nature of this disease and what one Nobel Prize winning medical professional believes is the root cause of this devastating illness.

Appendix VII:

Hydrogen Peroxide: Nature's Double-Edged Sword

From an atomic perspective, hydrogen peroxide (H_2O_2) is composed of four atoms, two each of both oxygen and hydrogen. Because this molecule is electrically unstable, the second oxygen atom is easily coaxed from this molecule resulting in two separate molecules: a water molecule (H_2O) and a singlet oxygen molecule (O_1). This change in physical configuration occurs in the presence of a variety of conditions including ultraviolet light, heat and the presence or organic matter.

The singlet oxygen molecule is a strong oxidizing agent. O_1 seeks electrical stability since it needs an additional electron to settle into a more stable state. One of the places it can get an electron is from an anaerobic micro-organism.

As it oxidizes these single cell organisms, the loss of electrons disorganizes their basic electrical cellular structures and functions and they die. Thus, hydrogen peroxide, as it breaks apart into its two component parts, actually becomes a very effective and relatively safe disinfectant.

The primary factor driving the growth in hydrogen peroxide consumption world-wide today is concern for the environment. Hydrogen peroxide naturally decomposes into two safe ingredients, water and oxygen. This makes hydrogen peroxide an excellent disinfectant as well as bleaching agent replacement for other very toxic oxidizing compounds like chlorine.

Until the early 1980s, hydrogen peroxide demand was equally distributed among pulp bleaching, chemical synthesis, disinfectant and the textile bleaching industries. Today, pulp bleaching accounts for over 67% of the demand for hydrogen peroxide in the U.S. and Canada and 48% of Western Europe's demand. The rapid growth for just this application alone has been driven by consumer pollution awareness and tighter governmental pollution regulations.

Only six companies have dominated the world hydrogen peroxide marketplace. They are, FMC Corporation (U.S.A., Degussa AG (Germany), DuPont (U.S.A.), Oxysynthese S.A. (France), and Mitsubishi Gas Chemical Company, Inc. (Japan). More recent entrants competing with these giants include Kemira Oy (Finland), Eka Nobel AB (Sweden) and Solvay Interox A.A. (owned by Solvay S.A. in Belgium). Solvay claims that it is the largest supplier of stabilized hydrogen peroxide for the cosmetic and food industries in the U.S.

There are six major grades of hydrogen peroxide based on the concentration of these molecules in water. These grades run from a low of three percent to a high of over 90%. They are:

(1) 3% H_2O_2 Used only for topical disinfecting. (This is the typical drug store variety.) This grade contains four or more toxic stabilizers to help reduce the molecular breakdown of the molecule to prevent the premature

release of oxygen. This grade is made using 50% super D peroxide and diluted to a three percent level.

(2) 6% H_2O_2: This is used primarily by beauticians for topical beaching of hair. It is available in a number of strengths and also contains toxic stabilizers.

(3) 30% Reagent H_2O_2: This grade is primarily used for medical research though it also contains toxic stabilizers.

(4) 30% - 32% Electronic Grade H_2O_2: This grade is used by the electronics' industry to wash transistors and integrated chips before assembly and contains toxic stabilizers.

(5) 35% Technical Grade H_2O_2: Used for a variety of scientific and industrial applications. This grade contains trace amounts of phosphorus and is used to counter-balance dissolved chlorine in water. This grade is not intended for human consumption.

(6) 35% Food Grade H_2O_2: Used for a variety of applications in the food preparation, food manufacturing and food packing industries, especially for cheese, whey and egg products. This grade is still very caustic and in this concentration can easily burn the skin. 35% food grade hydrogen peroxide must be diluted in order for it to be safe to handle, use and consume. *The F.D.A. has indicated that hydrogen peroxide is neither toxic nor carcinogenic. However, the F.D.A. strictly forbids the use of H2O2 for oxygen therapy usage.*

(7) 90% H_2O_2: This grade is used by N.A.S.A. as a fuel propellant oxygen source for the space program. This grade is extremely combustible and dangerous.

As you can see, the only hydrogen peroxide grade that can be used for human consumption is a dilution of 35% food grade. To be "safe", this grade should be diluted with water by at least 98%. Scientists and medical professionals now know that too much of the wrong kind of oxygen may be damaging to the body. While some hydrogen peroxide is naturally produced by the body's immune system and is broken down into its two component molecules by the enzyme catalase, too much H_2O_2 can produce an over abundance of singlet oxygen molecules (O_1) which can react with various components in the blood and cells to produce harmful free radicals.

Hydrogen peroxide oxygen therapies have been used for over 150 years with varying degrees of success. However, now that new and safer stabilized oxygen technologies exist, these new oxygen therapy technologies appear to be more preferable. More importantly, these new products do not require toxic stabilizers to insure that the molecules do not break down and prematurely release the oxygen.

As mentioned previously, "stabilized" hydrogen peroxide, like that purchased over-the-counter in brown bottles, contains stabilizers, like phosphoric acid, that are toxic. When other stable oxygen products are available that provide the same concentration of oxygen, this trade off for added shelf life hardly seems appropriate. Our goal should be to reduce, as far as possible, the ingestion or assimilation of carcinogenic or toxic materials.

Cosmetics and dental products, including tooth pastes, mouth washes, and gels, that claim they contain stabilized hydrogen peroxide may contain industrial or medical grade H2O2 that contains these toxic stabilizers. Putting this grade of peroxide on the skin or in the mouth, in any concentration, may actually be harming the body rather than bringing the body the added benefits of oxygenation. If the label does not state that food grade hydrogen peroxide is being used in its diluted form, then it would probably be advisable to refrain from using the product(s) until the actual contents are revealed.

As part of an alternative therapy, H2O2 is a double edged sword. While it can indeed help oxygenate the blood bringing countless benefits and relief from various diseases and ailments, it does have a darker side that can produce dangerous side effects. Many articles and books on the subject of H2O2 oxygen therapies fail to mention that extreme caution should be used whenever using peroxides for medicinal or preventative alternative therapies. In any case, individuals should consult with a qualified medical practitioner who has experience in a variety of oxygen therapies before personally using hydrogen peroxide for any protocol or to self-administer treatments for any ailment or condition.

Perhaps the insight and admonition of Dr. Cordel Logan, N.D., award-winning author of the book *Medicine at the Crossroads*, should be considered whenever administering hydrogen peroxide therapies. He wrote:

"Certainly excess hydrogen peroxide is harmful (may even aggravate Candida, cause rectal bleeding, and damage the digestive system)...Excessive hydrogen peroxide may inactivate adenylate cyclase (forms cyclic AMP), and cytochrome P-450 (a microsomal enzyme). It may inactivate SOD, rhodamese, trypsin, kinases, and other enzymes. Hydrogen peroxide inhibits immunoglobulins and causes red blood cell lysis (bursting)...Chromosomal damage has been reported. Dimethyl suloxide (DMSO), a scavenger for hydroxyl radicals, does not react with hydrogen peroxide or superoxide thus is not protective here...Extra hydrogen peroxide may combine with superoxide to form the hydroxyl radical which is a highly reactive free radical. This can cause peroxidation of unsaturated fatty acids. The healthy electrical charge from sialic acid can disappear leading to premature aging and other degenerative problems. (40)

As with many nutritional and alternative medicine approaches to health, too much of a "good thing" can be detrimental. Hydrogen peroxide, for nearly two centuries, has provided numerous health benefits. Caution, wisdom, and discernment as to the best approach to using H_2O_2 therapies should be the only approach to take.

For a more in-depth look at hydrogen peroxide and its use in oxygen therapies, please refer to the book written by Dr. Kurt Donsbach , D.C., Ph.D., entitled "Oxygen - Oxygen - Oxygen" In it, Dr. Donsbach discusses hydrogen peroxide, magnesium peroxide and chlorine peroxide. It is available directly from the Rockland Corporation (619-475-9951) or may be purchased at most health and nutrition stores.

Appendix VIII:

Oxygen Therapy: The First 150 Years

The following information is an edited version of the very detailed annotated chronology which was researched by Dr. Lawrence Martin, M.D., Chief, Division of Pulmonary and Critical Care Medicine at Mt. Sinai Medical Center, Cleveland, Ohio, U.S.A. A complete version may be obtained, free of charge, at the following website:

http://www.mtsinai.org/pulmonary/papers/ox-hist/ox-hist-intro.html.

Dr. Martin writes in his abstract's introduction: "Supplemental or 'extra' oxygen is one of the most widely used therapies for people admitted to the hospital. It is also frequently used for patients with chronic lung disease who live at home. In all cases, oxygen is administered by inhalation. The importance of oxygen therapy for many patients with heart and lung diseases is now universally recognized." (45)

An Oxygen Chronology from Priestly to Haldane Based Mainly on Original Sources

1772:   Swedish Apothecary Karl W. Scheele discovers "oxygen".

1774:   Chemist Joseph Priestly discovers oxygen simultaneously in England.

1775:   Joseph Priestly, LL.D.F.R.S. publishes "Experiments and Observations on Different Kinds of Air." Thomas Pearson, London MDCCXC (Three volumes published originally in 1775 and revised in 1790.)

1783   The first recorded treatment using oxygen therapies by French physician Calliens as published in the Gazette de Sante on a patient suffering from phthisis.

1789   The second recorded treatment using oxygen by French physician Chaptal of Montpellier for the same ailment.

1798   The Pneumatic Institution for inhalation and gas therapy was established by Thomas Beddoes, a British physician/philosopher, in Bristol. Quoted in the Bristol Gazette and Public Advertiser, March 21, 1799.

1820   Dr. Daniel Hill, M.D. publishes his pamphlet "Practical Observations on the Use of Oxygen, or Vital Air In the Cure of Diseases: To Which Are Added, a Few Experiments on the Vegetation of Plants, Illustrated with Five Engravings." Described are treatments for cases of nervous debility, epilepsy, hydrocephalus and scrophula as well as enhanced growth of plants exposed to oxygen.

1830   Dr. Benjamin Sillman, M.D. conducts a series of lectures on the benefits of oxygen therapies at Yale. The lectures: "Elements of Chemistry in the Order of Lectures Given in Yale College." New Haven; Printed and Published by Hezekiah Howe,, 1830.

1857   British doctor Dr. S.B. Birch, M.D. becomes a frequent contributor to British medical journals regarding the benefits of oxygen therapies. "On the Therapeutic Use of Oxygen." The Lancet, August 1, 1857.

1859   Dr. Birch publishes another article attributing cures to brief uses of oxygen inhalations. "On Oxygen as a Therapeutic Agent." British Medical Journal, December 24, 1859.

1866   French physician Dr. J.N. Demarquay publishes a 861 page compendium on the use of oxygen therapies by Europeans during the first few decades after its discovery as a gas. "Essay on Medical Pneumatology: A Physiological, Clinical and Therapeutic Investigation of the Gasses." Translated and published in 1889 with notes, additions by Dr. Samuel Wallian, A.M., M.D.

1869   Dr. Samuel S. Wallian, M.D. publishes his paper "Superoxygenation as a Therapeutic Measure" in the Chicago Medical Journal, February/March 1869.

1869   Dr. Edward Mackey publishes his paper "On the Therapeutical Value of the Inhalation of Oxygen Gas" in Pratitioner, Vol. 2, pgs. 276-287, 1869. Dr. Mackey cites 12 cases where treatments with oxygen demonstrated noted improvements in the patients.

1870   George Barth, inventor of "The Invalid's Oxygenator" and the patented "Oxygen Water" publishes a monograph, which includes information on his devices and case reports, entitled "Oxygen: A remedy in Disease." H.C. Balliere, 219 Regent Street, G. Barth, 36 Long Acre, W.C. 1870; 32 pages.

1870   Dr. Andrew H. Smith, M.D. publishes the prize-winning essay "Oxygen Gas as a Remedy in Disease." New York: D. Appleton & Company, 1870. Awarded the "Prize Essay of the Alumni Association of the College of Physicians and Surgeons, N.Y." This work is an extremely detailed description of the use of oxygen in clinical medicine at the time.

1872   Dr. J. Henry Davenport, M.D. publishes "Oxygen as a Remedial Agent" in the

Harvard Medical and Surgical Journal, July 25, 1872, Vol. X, No. 4, pgs. 61-64.

1881   Dr. G.R. Starkey, M.D. publishes his book "Compound Oxygen -- It's Mode of Action and Results", 1529 Arch Street, Philadelphia, 1881.

1885   Dr. Samuel S. Willian, M.D. publishes a follow-up paper entitled "Further Report: On Oxygen as a Therapeutic Agent." The Medical Record, October 31, 1885, pgs. 483-488.

1886   English physician Dr. Charles J. Smith, M.D., publishes the definitive paper on state-of-the-art 19th century oxygen therapies. "Clinical Notes: Oxygen in Therapeutics." Published in the Lancet, December 18, 1886, pg. 1172.

1887   A series of articles from Medical Current published in Chicago compiled by Dr. C.E. Ehinger, M.D. considered to be the most complete book on preparing and using medical oxygen at the time. "Oxygen in Therapeutics. A Treatise Explaining the Apparatus, the Material and the Processes Used in the Preparation of Oxygen and Other Gasses with which it May Be Combined; Also, It's Administration and Effects, Illustrated By Clinical Experience of the Author and Others." Chicago: W.A. Chatterhorn & Co., 1887.

1888   Dr. J.H. Kellogg, M.D., Superintendent of the Medical and Surgical Sanitarium at Battle Creek, MI, published an article discussing the benefits of alternative oxygen therapies. "Oxygen Enemata as a Remedy in Certain Diseases of the Liver and Intestinal Tract." Journal of the American Medical Association, 1888; 258-262.

1890   Dr. Albert Blodgett, M.D. publishes what is believed to be the first record documenting continuous oxygen therapy. "The Continuous Inhalation of Oxygen in Cases of Pneumonia Otherwise Fatal, and Other Diseases." Boston Medical and Surgical Journal (forerunner to the New England Journal of Medicine), Vol. CXXIII, No. 21, pgs. 481-484.

1908   Dr. William Seamann Bainbridge, M.D. publishes a review and brief history of oxygen therapies. "Oxygen in Medicine and Surgery -- A Contribution, with Report of Cases." New York State Journal of Medicine, Vol. 8, No. 6, June 1908, pgs. 281-295.

1910   Dr. W.H. Wilcox, M.D. and Professor B.J. Collingwood, M.D. (professor of Physiology, the Catholic University School of Medicine, Dublin, Ireland) reported on the benefits of oxygen mixed with alcohol for numerous physiological conditions. "The Therapeutic Use of Alcohol Vapour Mixed with Oxygen."

1914   Dr. H.O. Howitt, M.D., L.R.C.P., M.R.C.S. details the benefits of non-inhalation methods of giving oxygen. His report, along with those of Kellogg (1888), Bainbridge (1908) and Tunnicliffe & Stebbing (1916) highlights these new therapies for oxygen. "The Subcutaneous Injection of Oxygen Gas." The Canadian Medical Association Journal, 1914, Vol. 4; pgs. 983-985.

1916   Drs. F.W. Tunnicliffe, M.D. and G.F. Stebbing, M.D., both from London, investigate alternative methods of oxygen therapy other than inhalation. The Lancet, August 19, 1916; pgs. 321-323.

1917   Dr. J.S. Haldane, M.D. publishes his article on treating war gas injuries with oxygen therapies. "The Therapeutic Administration of Oxygen." F.R.S. British Medical Journal, February 10, 1917; pgs. 181-183.

1917   In America, the same year, Dr. S.J. Meltzer, M.D., LL.D. publishes what is considered one of the earliest articles on the therapeutic value of oxygen delivered under positive pressure. "The Therapeutic Value of Oral Rhythmic Insufflation of Oxygen." Journal of the American Medical Association, October 6, 1917; pgs. 1150-1156.

1920   A text of the discussions that took place on the therapeutic uses of oxygen on January 20th, 1920 under the direction of Drs. J. Barcroft, M.D. and J.S. Haldane, M.D. This is the first clear evidence that the science of oxygen therapies has taken hold instead of mere anecdotal reports and assumptions about the benefits of oxygen therapies. "Reports of Societies: Oxygen Therapy." Section of Therapeutics and Pharmacology of the Royal Science of Medicine. British Medical Journal, January 31, 1920.

Appendix IX:

Annotated Bibliography

For the most complete listing of articles on oxygen therapies, ozone and hydrogen peroxide, contact Dr. Gene Meyer, D.D.S. A biochemist, who has devoted much of his professional life to the study of oxygen and its effects on disease, Dr. Meyer has amassed one of the largest collections of oxygen-based literature in the U.S. today, almost 10,000 articles. His address is: 9725 E. Flower Street, Bellflower, CA 90706.

----

1.   Altman, Nathaniel. "Bio-Oxidative Therapy". Natural Health, November/December 1995: 44.

2.   Askew, Dr. Eldon W., Ph.D. "Environmental and Physical Stress and Nutrient Requirements." American Journal of Clinical Nutrition, 1995; 61 (Suppl.): 631S-7S. American Society for Clinical Nutrition.

3.   Ayur-Ved, Maharishi. Freedom from Disease: How to Control Free Radicals. Veda Publishing, Toronto, Canada: 1993.

4.   Baranowski, Zane. "Keep Breathing". Health Freedom News, October 1988: 31-34.

6.   Babior, B.M., 1982 "The Role of Active Oxygen in Microbial Killing by Phagocytes." In: Pathology of Oxygen, New York: Academic Press.

7. Berg, Dr. James D., Ph.D. "Technical Discussion: Stabilized Oxygen." Search For Health (U.S.A.), 1988.

8. Bio/Tech News. "Mighty 'Vitamin O'". Issue 16-B22, October 1997. Portland, OR.

9. Bland, Jeffrey S., Ph.D. "Age of the Virus". Delicious, November 1993: 40-43.

10. Bradford, R.W., Allen, H.W. and Culbert, M.L. Oxidology: The Study of Reactive Oxygen Toxic Species (ROTS) and their Metabolism in Health and Disease." The Robert W. Bradford Foundation, A Trust, Los Altos, CA (1985).

11. Braunwald, E. "Cyanosis, Hypoxia and Polycythemia", in Harrison's Principles of Internal Medicine. (7th Edition), McGraw, New York, 1974.

12. Bull, R.J., "Health Effects of Alternative Disinfectants and Their Reaction Products," J. AWWA, May: 229 (1980).

13. Bull, R.J., "Toxicological Problems Associated with Alternative Methods of Disinfection," J. AWWA Dec: 642 (1982).

14. Challem, Jack. "Are You Overdoing Antioxidants?" Natural Health, May/June 1995.

15. Challem, Jack. "Free Radicals and Antioxidants: A Contrarian View?" Nutrition Review, Natural Food Merchandiser Nutrition Science News, December 1995.

16. Cichoke, Dr. Anthony, M.A., D.C., D.A.C.B.N. "Inside/Out." The Energy Times, July/August 1994.

17. Cichoke, Dr. Anthony, M.A., D.C., D.A.C.B.N. "The Unsung Antioxidant: Zinc." Total Health, December 1993.

18. Donsbach, Kurt, N.D., Ph.D. Embracing Wholistic Health. Al-Don Institute of Experimental Medicine, Bonita, CA 1992: 61-62.

19. Donsbach, Kurt, N.D., Ph.D. Oxygen - Oxygen - Oxygen. Rockland Corporation: 1993; 13.

20. "Dinosaurs Weren't Done In By Asteroids", Associated Press Release, October 27, 1997.

21. Finn, Kathleen, "Antibiotics: Too Much of a Good Thing?" Delicious, October 1995: 30-34.

22. Gorner, Peter and Ronald Kotulak. "Scientists Try to Tame Molecular 'Sharks.'" Chicago Tribune, December 11, 1991.

23. Goulet, Brian. "Confessions of an Herbalist: The Magic of Aerobic Oxygen", Focus on Nutrition - The Canadian Journal of Health & Nutrition. (Issue No. 21), Burnaby, BC, 1989, Academic Press, N. Y., 1977.

24. Grim, Pamela, Lawrence Gottlieb, Allyn Boddie and Eric Batson. "Hyperbaric Oxygen Therapy". Journal of the American Medical Association, April 25, 1990, v. 263, n16: 2216(5).

25. Guyton, Arthur C. The Textbook of Medical Physiology, (5th Edition.) Pennsylvania:WB Saunders Co., 1976.

26. Halliwell, Dr. Barry, Ph.D. "Reactive oxygen species in living systems: source, biochemistry, and role in human disease." American Journal of Medicine, September 30, 1991, v91 n3C p14S(9).

27. International Association for Oxygen Therapy. A Divison of American Society of Medical Missionaries. P.O. Box 1360, Priest River, ID 83856. (208) 448-2657.

28. International Bio-Oxidative Medicine Foundation. P.O. Box 61767 Dallas/Ft. Worth, TX 75261. (817) 481-9772.

29. Jackson, William R., Ph.D. <u>Environmental Care & Share</u>. Jackson Research Center, 1995.

30. Jackson, William R., Ph.D. <u>Organic Soil Conditioning</u>. Jackson Research Center, 1993.

31. Korbakova, A.I. *Vestn. Akad. Med. Nauk.* 19:17 (1964).

32. Kugler, Dr. Hans, Ph.D. Preventative Medicine Update, March, 1988.

33. Lembreck, James, D.C.H., C.M.P. "Stabilized Oxygen...Breathe Easy". Natural Physique, June 1991: 85, 96.

34. Levine, Dr. Stephen. Biocurrents Press. Biocurrents Research and Development, Corporation. 944 Lake Street, San Francisco, CA, (415) 639-4575.

35. Levine, Dr. Stephen and Kidd, Dr. Parris. "Antioxidant Adaptation: It's Role in Free Radical Pathology." Biocurrents Press, San Francisco, 1987.

36. Levine, Dr. Stephen and Kidd, Dr. Parris. 1985, "Beyond Anti-Oxidant Adaptation: A Free Radical-Hypoxia-Clonal Thesis of Cancer Causation," J. Orthomol. Medicine, 14(3):189-213.

37. Levine, Dr. Stephen. <u>Biocurrents Press</u>. Biocurrents Research and Development, Corporation. 944 Lake Street, San Francisco, CA, (415) 639-4575.

38. Levine, Dr. Stephen and Kidd, Dr. Parris. "Antioxidant Adaptation: It's Role in Free Radical Pathology." <u>Biocurrents Press</u>, San Francisco, 1987.

39. Levine, Dr. Stephen and Kidd, Dr. Parris M. (co-authors): "Antioxidant Adaptation" and

"Immunity, Cancer, Oxygen, and Candida Albicans". <u>Let's Live</u>, August, 1986.

40. Logan, Cordell, Ph.D., N.D. <u>Medicine at the Crossroads</u>, Logan Press, Logan, UT (1993)

41. Lubbers, J.R., J.R. Bianchine, and R.J. Bull, "Safety of Oral Chlorine Dioxide, Chlorite, and Chlorate Ingestion in Man." Ch. 95, pp 1335-1341 in R.L. Jolley, Ed. <u>Water Chlorination: Environmental Impact and Health Effects</u>, Vol. 4 Ann Arbor Science, Ann Arbor, MI (1982).

42. McCabe, Ed. <u>Oxygen Therapies: A New Way of Approaching Diseases</u>. Energy Publications, Morrisville, NY (1994).

43. McAllister Smart. "Antioxidants for the Uninitiated." Vegetarian Times, April 1994.

44. McCord, Joe and Findivich, Irwin. <u>Superoxides and Superoxide Dismutases</u>. Academic Press, N. Y., 1977. McGaffigan, Patricia A., R.N., M.S. "Hazards of Hypoxemia," Nursing, May, 1996.

45. Martin, Dr. Lawrence, M.D. "Oxygen Therapy: The First 150 Years". Abstract. Mt. Sinai Medical Center, Cleveland, Ohio. Internet File. February, 1997.

46. Masschelein, W.J. and Rice, Rip G. <u>Chlorine Dioxide: Chemistry and Environmental Impact of Oxychlorine Compounds</u>. Ann Arbor Science Publishers, Inc., Ann Arbor, MI.

47. Morales, Betty Lee. "The Free Radical -- The Common Denominator of Disease." Let's Live, July 1982.

48. Muntz, John, D.O., Ph.D. "The Case for Stabilized Oxygen". Health World, August 1991: 12.

299

49. Neergaard, Lauren. "Battling the SUPERBUG". Telegram Tribune, Science/Environment, Feb, 24, 1996: E-8.

50. Paulet, G. and S. Desbrousser. <u>Arch. Mal. Prof</u>. 33:59 (1972), 31:97 (1970) and 35:797 (1974).

51. Pizzorno, Joseph E., N.D. "Neutrophil Power". Natural Health, Sept/Oct 1994: 82-83, 125-130

52. Priestley, Joseph, LL.D.F.R.S. Experiments and Observations on Different Kinds of Air and Other Branches of Natural Philosophy Connected with the Subject (in three volumes). Printed by Thomas Pearson and Sold by J. Johnson, St. Paul's Church-Yard, London. MDCCXC.

53. Robbins, John. <u>Diet for a New America</u>. Stillpoint Publishing, New Hampshire, 1987.

54. Rothchild, Peter. <u>Enzyme Therapy in Immune Complex and Free Radical Contingent Diseases</u>. University Lab Press, Hawaii, 1988.

55. Rothshild, Peter R. and Fahey, William. <u>Free Radicals, Stress and Antioxidant Enzymes</u>. University Labs Press, Honolulu, HI: 1991; 3-4.

56. Sevy, Jonathan B., D.C. "Drugs, Not Foods, Are Toxic." Dynamic Chiropractic. December 17, 1993.

57. Smith, Dr. Andrew H., M.D. Oxygen Gas As a Remedy In Disease. New York: D. Appleton & Company, 1870.

58. Starr, Sonya C., B.S., N.C. "Oxygen -- O2: The Life Giving Element." The Nutrition & Dietary Consultant, August 1986.

59. Sweet, F. et al. "Ozone Selectivity Inhibits the Growth of Human Cancer Cells." <u>Science</u>: 209:931 (1980).

60. Thompson, Donald C., M.D. "Invisible Toxins Hurt the Immune System." Journal of Longevity Research, Vol3, No. 5, 1997: 26-27.

61. Walker, Dr. Morton, D.P.M. "Fruit & Vegetable Antioxidants: New Research." Health Food Business, July 1995.

62. Warburg, O., 1969, The Prime Cause and Prevention of Cancer, (1966 Lindau Lecture, English Edition by D. Burke), Wurzburg, Germany: K. Trilsch.

63. Warburg, O., 1966, The Lindau Lecture. Germany.

64. West, C. Samuel. The Golden Seven Plus One, (Seventh Printing), Utah: Samuel Publishing, April 1988.

65. ----- "Exotic diseases are sounding alarms", Washington (AP), Telegram Tribune, Jan. 3, 1995; 1.

66. ----- "Why antibiotics are failing to protect us from seemingly common viruses and what you can do to protect yourself." Energy Times, March 1996: 29-33.

67. ----- "Staph germ becoming unstoppable", Telegram Tribune, Tues. May 29, 1997: 1.

Appendix X:

Oxygen & Nutritional Glossary

- A -

Acid-Alkaline Balance: The body's pH, a measurement of the body's acidity or alkalinity, is 80% alkaline and 20% acidic by design. Most diets, even those of vegetarians, are 75% acidic and 25% alkaline. Excesses in either area result in a lack of hydrochloric acid (HCl) in the stomach which reduces the production of pancreatic enzymes that are important in the digestion process. As the food sits in the stomach and the intestines undigested or partially digested it ferments (rots).

This putrid mass will travel through almost 40 feet of intestines spreading toxic poisons. There will be a resulting poor assimilation of nutrients from the consumed foods and an increase of toxins in the blood stream.

Coffee, tea, soft drinks and other foods radically alter the body's pH to the acidic side. A highly acidic body will provide an environment where yeasts, viruses, parasites and cancer cells thrive. In addition, bodies that suffer acidic states for prolonged periods consume the body's stored reserves of sodium, calcium, potassium and magnesium. This reserve of minerals is crucial for acting as catalysts that activate the enzymes that digest and assimilate food.

Aerobic: A condition or state that contains oxygen. Aerobic organisms are ones that can only survive (live) and only reproduce in an oxygen-rich environment or atmosphere. The opposite state or condition is called "anaerobic".

Amino Acid: The basic building block used by every cell in the body to manufacture proteins. What distinguishes one protein from another is the way the cells assemble amino acids into proteins. There are over 20 different amino acids that combine in different ways and combinations to make all of the proteins we need to grow. These proteins are divided into two groups: essential amino acids, (there are eight of these that cannot be manufactured by the body and must be derived from the foods we eat,) and non-essential amino acids, (there are twelve of these and they are manufactured by the body.)

Anabolism: The chemical process in the body where a more complex substance is built from simpler ones. This process requires energy which cannot happen without the presence of oxygen. An example of an anbolic process is the synthesis of proteins from amino acids.

Anaerobic: A condition or state that lacks oxygen. Almost all pathogenic (harmful) organisms that cause disease are anaerobic. These include bacteria, viruses, yeasts, molds, fungi and parasites. When these organisms are placed in an oxygen-rich state or atmosphere, these organisms die.

Anion: A negatively charged ion. (See "ion.")

Antibiotics: An anti-bacterial substance used against an organisms created from or out of another living organism. Penicillin is a relatively non-toxic acidic substance extracted from the green mold Penicillun notatum that has very powerful anti-bacterial properties.

Antioxidant: A group of vitamins, minerals and enzymes that the body uses to protect itself against the formation of free radicals. (See "free radicals".) Antioxidant molecules include vitamins A, C, E, the B-family, gamma-linoleic acid (GLA) and L-cysteine.

Artery: One of the main tubular-shaped branching vessels from the heart that carries the oxygen and nutrient-rich blood to the organs and cells in the body.

Arthritis: An inflammation of a joint in the body associated with pain, swelling, stiffness and redness. It is believed that arthritis is caused by bacterial infections. Oxygen therapies are the newest approach to relieving both the symptoms and the cause of most types of arthritis.

A.T.P. (Adenosine Tri-Phosphate): This chemical compound, comprised of carbon, hydrogen, nitrogen, oxygen and phosphorus, is the essential by-product of the combination of oxygen and glucose in the cells. A.T.P. is the "energy pack" used for cellular metabolism. Without A.T.P., the cells cannot create heat nor can they function properly.

- B -

Bacteria: A large group of primarily one-celled microorganisms from the class Schizomycetes that are usually parasitic or saprophytic (living on dead or decaying matter). Bacteria are spherical in shape (coccus), rod-shaped (bacillus) or spiral or thread-like shaped (spirillum). Many bacteria cause diseases like food poisoning and pneumonia, while others are very active in food fermentation and the conversion of dead organic matter into nutrients for plants.

Basophils: Basophils are white blood cells that function as the signal core to let the immune system know that heparin needs to be released into the blood stream. Heparin is the substance that prevents the blood from coagulating. Heparin also functions as a substance that removes fat (cholesterol) particles from the blood stream.

Bilirubin: Bilirubin is the waste product of the decomposition and breakdown of red blood cells and hemoglobin. Bilirubin is transported by the body to the liver where it is converted to bile.

Blood: In mammals, blood is usually a deep red, sticky fluid that circulates through the thousands of miles of veins, arteries and capillaries in the body. Blood is manufactured in the marrow of bones. Blood's main function is to serve as the body's transportation system for nutrients, oxygen and wastes from cellular metabolism. It is called the "river of life" because within this ever flowing river is everything the body needs to sustain itself and also fight off disease. Almost 95% of the blood is actually a somewhat clear, slightly saline (salty) liquid called the "plasma". The blood also contains three types of blood cells: the red blood cells (erethrocytes), white blood cells (leukocytes) and platelets (thrombocytes). Each of these blood cells has a specific and important function to maintain life.

- C -

Cancer: A disease whereby normal, healthy cells alter their metabolic functioning from aerobic (respiration) to anaerobic (fermentation). Researchers now believe that cancer develops when the body has been deprived for long periods of an adequate supply of oxygen (hypoxemia). The scientific evidence strongly suggests that, unlike normal cells in the body, cancer cells thrive in a low-body oxygen state. As far back as 1956, Nobel prize winner Dr. Otto Warburg found that chemicals accumulating in the tissues of the body cause 80% of all cancers. (See Appendix VI for a complete text of Dr. Warburg's discussion of his cancer research.)

Candida: Candida (short for Candida albicans) is a small, oval-shaped budding fungus that causes mycotic infections in both men and women. Normally, Candida infects the digestive tract but can spread throughout the entire body resulting in systemic infection. Candida is usually controlled by the friendly, aerobic bacteria Acidophilus that consumes Candida as a Primary food source.

If allowed to grow out of control, Candida can produce significant amounts of toxins as part of the waste product of the yeast's metabolic cycle. These toxins cause fatigue, dizziness, constipation, diarrhea, cramping, etc.

Candida infections can also result in liver damage as well as damage to the nervous system. Candida can impair the immune and circulatory systems and suppress hormone production in women.

Most physicians continue to treat Candida (vaginal yeast) infections in women with medications (drugs) that suppress the symptoms but do not stop the cause. Candida thrives on carbohydrates, sugar yeasts and fermented foods in a low oxygen environment in the body.

Many individuals who suffer the symptoms of Candida infections do not realize they are infected with this yeast and are feeding it every day with the foods they eat.

Stabilized oxygen and other oxygen therapies have proved to be a very natural and successful alternative therapy to traditional drugs in controlling and eliminating Candida infections.

Capillaries: The smallest blood vessels that deliver oxygen to the cells. If capillaries become clogged or damages, vital nutrients cannot be delivered to the cells resulting in diminished cellular health. Cells starved of oxygen for prolonged periods of time either die or, as described by Nobel Prize winner Dr. Otto

Warburg, their metabolism changes and the cells become cancerous.

Carbohydrates: A group of substances that provide the body with one of its two main sources of energy. (The other group is fats). There are three main types of carbohydrates: monosaccharides (which include sucrose, galactose and fructose,) disaccharides (which include sucrose, lactose and maltose,) and polysaccharides (which include starch and cellulose). Oxygen combines with glucose, the simplest form of sugar derived from carbohydrates to create the energy needed for all cellular metabolic functions. The body will break down all complex carbohydrates into glucose and glycogen. (Glycogen is stored as an energy reserve fuel in fat cells.)

Carbon Dioxide: Carbon dioxide (CO_2) is the main waste product of cellular metabolism. It is created when glucose is combined with oxygen to make energy for the cell. After the red blood cells release their life-giving oxygen to the cells, the hemoglobin receptors pick up the the CO_2 to return these molecules to the lungs where they can be expelled.

Carcinogen: Carcinogens are substances or stress states that prevent the body from producing metabolic energy and which facilitate in the rise of cancerous cell growth. These stress states can be physical, electrical or psychological in nature. Physical factors include pollutants (such as tobacco tars, unsaturated oils, carbon monoxide, chemical additives to foods, etc.) Electrical factors include excessive exposure to X-rays, microwaves, fluorescent lights, radio waves and ultra-violet light. Electrical signals can destroy critical chemical bonds within the cells. Psychological factors include prolonged stress which drains the body of nutrients and energy and weakens the immune system.

Catabolism: The process whereby the body breaks down complex substances into simpler components that the body can use for normal metabolism. Glycogen, a more complex sugar (carbohydrate), is catabolized into glucose, the simplest sugar, which is combined with oxygen in the cells to produce energy.

Cation: A positively charged (+) ion. Cations get their name from the fact that during the electrolysis process, these ions travel in the solution to the positively charged cathode. (See "ion".)

Cell: The basic and most simplest living unit of our bodies. Every organ is an aggregate of millions of living cells held together by a supporting foundation called "intercellular supporting structures." Every cell,. regardless of where it is in the body, has a specific function. All cells must have a sufficient supply of oxygen to combine with carbohydrates, fats and/or proteins to release energy for cellular functions. It is estimated that we have 25 trillion red blood cells and 75 million other cells in our bodies. Whenever a cell is damaged or destroyed, the surrounding cells usually generate new cells until the appropriate number of cells are present.

Chemotherapy: A traditional medical procedure whereby extremely toxic drugs are used to kill cancer cells. Unfortunately, these drugs are not selective and have significant side effects on normal tissues. Chemotherapy drugs reduce or destroy the cell's ability to reproduce itself. These drugs affect the bone marrow and halt the production of both red and white blood cells. Chemotherapy drugs also affect the intestinal lining, the hair follicles, the mouth and other organs.

Chloride: A compound in which chlorine has combined with another substance, usually minerals like sodium, magnesium, potassium, etc. Chloride, as a negatively charged ion (Cl-), is a very important part of the body's metabolic cycle and is recognized by the F.D.A. as an essential nutrient for the body.

Chlorine: Both the proper chemical name as well as the description of a class of highly toxic and carcinogenic gas that is easily dissolved in water. Chlorine gas is a deadly killer of pathogenic microbes but it also reacts with humic acid in the body to form trihalomethane (like chloroform) which is suspected of causing numerous degenerative diseases. Chlorine, when it has lost an electron and is bound to certain minerals, forms a chloride ion. Chloride is an essential part of the body's metabolic cycle.

Chlorine Dioxide (Chlorite): Chlorine dioxide (ClO_2), also called "chlorite", is created when chlorine atoms combine with oxygen to form a relatively stable oxy-halogen molecule. Chlorite is a very strong oxidizing agent and is used in the paper and tanning industry as a bleaching agent. Chlorine dioxide is also used to purify (disinfect) waste water as a substitute for chlorine. In the last 10 years it has become popular as a stabilized oxygen dietary supplement competing with hydrogen peroxide. Caution should be used when consuming chlorite as it is typically quite alkaline and can burn the skin, eyes, and delicate membranes in the mouth, esophagus, and respiratory tract. Most chlorine dioxide supplements require the product to be diluted before consumption.

Circulatory System: This is the blood's "highway" in the body. The circulatory system is broken down into two systems which describe the direction of the blood flow. The systemic circulatory system is the system that supplies oxygen-rich blood to the entire body, except the lungs, and then returns the blood back to the lungs to release carbon dioxide. The circulatory system includes the aorta (the body's main artery), arterioles (smaller arteries), capillaries, veins and venules (smaller veins).

Veins are very different than arteries because they have one-way valves that prevent the blood from flowing backward and are arranged in the body so that the blood flow can only be in one direction towards the heart. The circulatory system also takes a detour to the liver (called the portals circulatory system). This is where capillaries carrying nutrient-rich blood from the stomach, intestines and other digestive organs all meet together in one place. The liver then processes these nutrients, stores them, or allows them to pass back into the systemic circulatory system.

The second part of the circulatory system is the pulmonary circulatory system which is solely responsible for re-oxygenating the blood and serves as the source of oxygen and nutrients for the lungs.

Coenzyme Q10: This enzyme, manufactured in our bodies, works along side of other enzymes to support the body's bio-energetic functions. Coenzyme Q10 appears to be a mild immune system stimulant and research indicates that this enzyme affects the heart's pumping action as well as its electrical functioning. It is also believed that coenzyme Q10 lowers blood pressure.

Colostrum: Colostrum is considered to be Nature's perfect food. It is the "pre-milk" or "first milk" substance produced in the breasts by all mammals during the first 24 hours of lactation. Colostrum provides the infant with immune and growth hormone factors and the perfect combination of vitamins, minerals, amino acids and proteins to insure the health, vitality and growth of a newborn.

Bovine (cow) colostrum contains higher levels of all vital nutrients than human colostrum and is harvested under strict F.D.A. and U.S.D.A. guidelines for use as a human dietary supplement. When taken orally or topically, colostrum is very beneficial in strengthening the immune system of in fighting off illness.

- D -

Digestive System: The digestive system is designed to break food down into its basic chemical components, (vitamins, minerals, amino acids, proteins, sugars, etc.) These component molecules can then be absorbed into the blood stream and used for the metabolic processes of the cells and organs. The digestive tract consists of the mouth, pharynx, esophagus, stomach, intestines, duodenum, jejunum, ileum, cecum, colon, rectum and anus. The associated digestive organs include the salivary glands, liver and pancreas.

Disease: A condition where the body's health is in jeopardy. Disease is caused primarily because of a lack of cellular oxygen, the inability of the cell to use oxygen, a lack or an excess of nutrients, or the body's inability to control or eliminate wastes or toxic substances.

D.S.H.E.A.: The Dietary and Supplement Health Education Act (D.S.H.E.A.) was passed by congress in 1996 and went into law on January 1, 1997. The F.D.A. attempted to control and regulate dietary supplements under pressure from the medical and pharmaceutical industries. In response to the F.D.A.'s proposals, consumers all over the country reacted and forced legislators to protect their rights to choose alternative nutritional approaches without restrictions from the government. This law defines the classification of dietary supplements as well as government's limited role in regulating these nutritional items.

- **E** -

Electrolyte: A substance that disassociates (breaks down) into ions when fused or when dissolved in a solution and thus will conduct electricity. Within the body, electrolytes play an essential role in the structure and working of every cell as well as maintaining fluid and acid-base balance. The most important electrolytes are: (1) sodium, a key water-balance regulator and necessary for the normal functioning of both muscles and nerves; (2) potassium, associated with acid-base balance and the main constituent of cytoplasm in the cells; (3) calcium, important for blood clotting and for normal muscle physiology; (4) magnesium and chloride, essential for the chemical changes required for all body functions.

Electron: An extremely small part of each atom associated with the atom's electrical field or charge. An abundance of electrons surrounding an atom leads to a negative charge, a lack of electrons results in a positive charge. Electrons circle the nucleus of an atom in orbits.

Emphysema: A chronic obstructive pulmonary disease (COPD) that affects the lung tissue and prevents oxygen from being transferred into the blood stream. Since 1982, diseases of the lungs in the U.S. alone has increased more than 40%. It is now the fourth leading cause of death in the U.S. killing over 85,000 people each year. The main reason for this increase is the rise of cigarette smoking among Americans after World War II. Research clearly shows that smoking causes emphysema in over 80% of all individuals who do smoke.

The chemicals, gasses and tars in tobacco smoke block the production of a necessary protein called alpha1-antitrypsin (AAT). Loss of AAT's protection allows other enzymes to destroy the elastic fibers in the air sacs in the lungs. Now, fifty years after the end of the war, smoking's progressive lung destruction is taking its toll.

Other causes of emphysema include prolonged exposure to industrial fumes, (especially those from coal mines and rock quarries,) and exposure to high levels of smog.

Endocrine System: The endocrine system is a collection of glands which produce hormones. Hormones regulate metabolism, growth and sexual development. The main glands that make up this system are: (1) the pituitary gland, which stimulates the adrenals, thyroid and gonads as well as affects skin pigmentation and growth hormones; (2) the thyroid gland, which stimulates metabolism, body heat production and bone growth; (3) the parathyroid gland, which regulates the levels of calcium in the blood; (4) the adrenal glands, which when stimulated by the pituitary glands maintain the blood pressure and the salt balance of the body; (5) the pancreas, which secretes insulin and glucagon which controls the use of glycogen for cell energy production; (6) the ovaries, which produce estrogen and progesterone and thus influence female physiology; (7) the testes which produce testosterone that stimulates sperm production and the development of male physiology.

Enzyme: Stamina, energy levels and the strength of the immune system are directly related to the level of enzymes in the body. As we get older, the levels of enzymes decrease and disease gains a stronger foothold. Enzymes are complex organic compounds that accelerate (catalyze) the transformation of other substances in the body into substances that the body can use for metabolism. There are three types of enzymes: (1) digestive enzymes, which are secreted by the pancreas, stomach and small intestines; (2) food enzymes, which we obtain from raw, uncooked fruits, vegetables, sprouts, soaked seeds and nuts -- cooking destroys these enzymes; (3) metabolic enzymes, which regulate the functions of the blood, tissues and organs. Vitamins and minerals cannot be used by the body unless the proper enzymes are present.

E.P.A.: Environmental Protection Agency. A U.S. governmental regulatory agency originally established to monitor water and air quality to protect citizens from pollution.

Eosinophils: Esinophils are white blood cells that play an important role in reducing the contaminations in the blood stream that cause allergic reactions. They are also present in increased numbers whenever the body is suffering from parasitic infestation.

Essential Mineral: It is foolish to believe that the foods we consume today supply all of the nutrients essential to optimum health. Foods of all kinds are the end product of over-processed manufacturing and preparation and have been stripped of vital nutrients, especially vitamins and minerals, which are essential for normal body functions. The federal government has established the recommended daily allowance (RDA) for minerals to maintain normal health. These essential minerals include selenium, magnesium, calcium, zinc, iron, sodium and potassium.

Extracellular Fluid: This is the fluid in the spaces outside or surrounding the cells. Cells are considered to be in a "dry state" when there is only enough extracellular fluid to fill the small spaces and crevices between each cell. Edema is the condition where there is too much fluid between the cells. This excess fluid can choke the cells and cause pressure damage to the blood vessels and nerves.

- **F** -

Fats: Fats provide the body with the most concentrated form of fuel energy. Fats consist of fatty acids which contain carbon, hydrogen and very few oxygen atoms. Fats fall into two main groups: saturated and unsaturated. Saturated fatty acids contain the highest concentration of hydrogen atoms and are the basic components of meat and dairy products. Unsaturated fats are those that do not contain a complete or full bonding of hydrogen atoms at each of the available receptor sites on the molecules. Vegetable fats (oils) are unsaturated fats.

F.D.A.: The U.S. Food and Drug Administration. The F.D.A. is a federal regulatory agency that controls the pharmaceutical, food production, food processing, food supplement and drug industries in the U.S. The F.D.A.'s powers are sweeping and control every area of the health care profession, including hospitals, physicians, medical equipment, therapies, nutritional, over-the-counter drugs, etc.

Free Radical: Unstable atoms or groups of atoms that can cause damage to our cells, impair our immune system and can eventually lead to infections and various degenerative diseases are called free radicals. Free radicals have both beneficial functions in attacking pathogenic microbes in the body as well as a cumulative detrimental affect. There are three well-documented groups of free radicals: the superoxide, the hydroxyl and the peroxide.

Any of these may be formed by exposure to radiation, toxic chemicals, over-exposure to ultraviolet light, or as a result of metabolic processes including the conversion of fat molecules into simpler sugars for fuel for energy. Free radicals are kept in check naturally in the body by free radical scavengers which neutralize the free radicals as they are produced.

Four key enzymes function in this way. They are superoxide dismutase (SOD), methione reductase, catalase and glutathione peroxidase. All are produced as needed by a healthy body. In addition, other antioxidants include the vitamins A, E, C, the B family and the mineral selenium. (See Chapter 5 and Appendix IV for more details on free radicals.)

Fungus (Fungi): In human physiology, fungi are a group of living plants, unicellular or multi-cellular in form, that are devoid of chlorophyll and reproduce by means of releasing spores. Fungi live off of dead or decaying matter. In some cases, where the surface (skin) cells have become diseased, damaged or the health has been impaired, pathogenic fungi can find a host medium and thus thrive.

- G -

Glucose: A simple sugar ($C_6H_{12}O_6$) which is absolutely critical in the production of energy in every living cell in the body. Glucose is combined with oxygen in the cell to produce A.T.P. (see "A.T.P.") which is the energy source for cellular metabolism.

Glycogen: A more complex sugar (starch) than glucose that is usually stored in either the liver or in fat cells. Glycogen is the energy reserve fuel for the body. As glucose is depleted, the body draws on this reserve and breaks down the glycogen molecule into glucose which the cells can then use to produce energy.

Granulocyte: A family of white blood cells that include neutrophils, basophils and eosinophils. Also called "polymorphonuclear leukocytes", they are called granulocytes because the cells look like they are filled with small granules when viewed under a microscope.

- H -

Hemoglobin: Hemoglobin is the respiratory pigment in each red blood cell. Hemoglobin's main component is iron and hemoglobin's main function is to react with oxygen from the lungs to form oxyhemoglobin. This new molecule is then transported through the blood stream to the capillaries where it is released for the cells to use for respiration and metabolism. Once hemoglobin releases its oxygen molecule, it picks up carbon dioxide and transports this waste gas back to the lungs where it is replaced with another oxygen molecule.

Holistic: In 1926, the South African philosopher, Jan Christian Smuts originated the concept "holistic" to mean whole. Many today refer to holistic as "wholistic" and use the terms interchangeably to mean "whole" "holy" and "healthy". At the basis of holistic medicine is the fact that each of us is responsible for our own health and that preventing disease and sickness is far better than fighting off illness. The goal is "wellness" not just the absence of disease. Physicians and health practitioners are "partners" in maintaining a healthy body, mind and spirit.

Homeopathy: The term "homeopathy" comes from the Greek words "homeosis", meaning similar, and "pathos", meaning suffering or sickness. Homeopathy is thus an alternative approach to health based on the law of similars, or as Hippocrates wrote, "like cures like". Homeopathic remedies contain small doses of natural substances that come from plants, animals and/or minerals that normally would cause illness or a physiological reaction if taken in larger amounts. The alternative approach works by stimulating the body's own natural defenses and allowing the body to heal itself and helping the body to maintain a natural balance. In traditional medicine, an allergy or flu shot is a homeopathic remedy for preventing disease.

Hormones: A group of chemicals, produced by the organs, (a gland or tissue,) and released into the blood stream that has a specific and unique effect on tissues or organs somewhere else in the body. Hormones control a variety of body functions including growth, response to illness, stress and disease, as well as sexual development. The more important hormone producing glands and tissues include the adrenal glands, gonads, pancreas, thyroid, parathyroid, pituitary and placenta. The kidneys, brain and intestines also secrete hormones.

Hydrogen Peroxide: Hydrogen peroxide ($H2O2$) is merely a water molecule that has an added oxygen molecule attached to it ($H2O + O1 \implies H2O2$). Hydrogen peroxide is reported to have excellent oxygenating and oxidizing qualities for use in a variety of applications including disinfecting, cosmetics and oxygen therapies. Hydrogen peroxide is also naturally produced by the body as an instrumental part of the immune system's defense mechanisms against invading pathogens. Hydrogen peroxide is also a key ingredient in colostrum, the first milk consumed by infants. (See Appendix VII.)

Hypoxemia: The condition where there is a less than adequate supply of oxygen for the cells and tissues of the body which predisposes an individual to a number of degenerative diseases including circulatory problems, digestive disorders and even cancer. When insufficient oxygen is available in the body and blood stream, carbon monoxide (CO) is formed and is not easily eliminated. CO forms a very strong bond with hemoglobin and is not easily displaced by O2. Thus the level of available oxygen declines preventing the cells from producing the energy necessary for healthy metabolism.

Toxins begin to build up, organs get irritated, the body temperature is reduced, and bacteria and viruses gain a stronger foothold in the low oxygen environment. Individuals suffering from hypoxemia report symptoms like increased headaches, dizziness, insomnia, constipation, faintness, loss of appetite, heart palpitations, impaired kidney functions, cold hands and feet, impaired gland functions and a variety of lymphatic and blood disorders. Oxygen therapies can help bring back the oxygen levels in the body to more normal levels.

- ▮ -

Immune System: The body's immune system consists of over one trillion white blood cells (lymphocytes) and

100 million molecules called antibodies that are produced and secreted by these lymphocytes. These cells and antibodies find their way into every cell and every space in the body to help protect the body from bacteria, fungi, viruses, parasites, yeasts, molds and even cancer cells during our lifetime. To be "immune" is to be protected, to have resistance, to be exempt from disease. The immune system also includes the skin, which acts as a barrier against disease, the bone marrow, which produces white blood cells, the thymus, spleen, lymph nodes, adenoids and the digestive tract. Oxygen is a key ingredient to a healthy immune system. The lack of oxygen reduces the immune system's ability to fight off disease.

Intracellular Fluid: This is the fluid that is inside every cell. It contains high amounts of potassium, magnesium and phosphate ions and smaller amounts of sodium and chloride ions.

Ion: An electrically charged atom or groups of atoms. Some compounds, like salts, acids and bases, are thought to consist wholly or partly of ions held together by electrical attraction. During the electrolysis process, (a process that is used to make almost all stabilized oxygen solutions today,) negative ions ("anions"), which contain an excess of one or more electrons and are presented by a negative sign "-" after their chemical symbols, always move towards the anode. The positive ions ("cations"), which are missing one or more electrons and are represented by a positive sign "+" after their chemical symbols, always move towards the cathode. In gasses, a molecule can lose an electron and become a positive ion and the free electron may attach itself to another molecule or atom and become a negative ion.

- K -

Kidneys: The kidneys influence and control both body fluids and numerous nutrients that the body requires for metabolism. The kidneys regulate and filter the blood, control electrolytes (like sodium and potassium), regulate the pH of the body to keep the body from becoming too acidic or alkaline, control the amount of water in the body, help eliminate waste products, and produce several very important hormones, especially the ones that help regulate the Production and the release of red blood cells.

- L -

Liver: The liver is the largest and certainly one of the most important organs in the body. It is the main chemical production factory in the body and has five main functions: (1) the production of proteins, including albumin, complement, coagulation factors and globin; (2) the control of glucose by storing extra glucose as glycogen; (3) the control of amino acids; the filtering of poisonous drugs and substances from the blood; (5) the production of bile which carries away wastes and helps in the breakdown and absorption of fats in the small intestine.

Lymphatic (Lymph) System: The volume of the lymphatic system exceeds that of the blood in our bodies. While blood is a carrier of nutrients, lymph actually nourishes the cells. It is designed to filter out of the body large molecules, like bacteria and toxins. Approximately 90% of the fluids in the body pass through the capillaries. The remaining 10%, which includes dead cells and small particles, is transported to the heart through the lymphatic system. This system is remarkable because of its one-way valves called "lymph nodes". These nodes trap micro-organisms and foreign bodies. The specialized white blood cells that reside in the nodes (lymphocytes) neutralize and destroy invading pathogens. The lymph constantly circulates through this system. This lymph liquid is moved along by muscle action and not by the pressure created by the pumping of the heart.

Lymphocytes: Lymphocytes are a type of white blood cell that are formed in the lymph glands instead of the bone marrow. These cells travel between the blood stream, lymph glands and the channels between the lymph glands. While there are a number of differentiated lymphocytes, the two most important types are the T-type and the B-type. T-cells are called "killer" white blood cells because they are responsible for attacking abnormal cells in the body, like cancer cells. B-type lymphocytes are responsible for forming antibodies that protect the body against a second attack from diseases that previously found a foothold in the body and that the body was able to defend itself against. These "B-type" cells form an integral part of the immune system.

- M -

Magnesium: One of the most important minerals in the body and found in over 300 different enzymes that the body uses. It is critically important in the process of creating energy in the cells which involves its combination with glucose and oxygen. Most of the magnesium in the body is used in our bone structure and is actively involved in cellular metabolism. Correct magnesium levels in the body helps protect the body against heart disease, hypoglycemia, reduces kidney stone formation and reduces the severity of P.M.S. A lack of magnesium results in cramping, poor appetite, diarrhea, mental instability, confusion or forgetfulness and even convulsions.

Magnesium Peroxide: A molecule in which the mineral magnesium, an essential mineral in the body, is bonded to two oxygen atoms forming the chemical combination MgO_2. Magnesium peroxide's molecular bonding between the magnesium and oxygen atoms can be broken by numerous acids, (like citric and hydrochloric acids,) and thus releases the diatomic oxygen molecule (O_2) for the body to use in its metabolic processes. Magnesium peroxide has been used as a body oxygenator.

M.D.R. (Minimum Daily Requirement): Originally, the M.D.R. was established by the federal government to prevent acute diseases in animals and initiated during

World War II. Today, the Federal Drug Administration (F.D.A.) has established the minimum daily amount of nutrients it recommends to maintain a modecum of average health. These minimums include carbohydrates, proteins, etc. (Also see R.D.A.)

Metabolism/Metabolic Cycle: The chemical changes in living cells which provide for the cells' vital process and activities is called the cells' "metabolic cycle". All these functions require the production and use of energy. At the heart of energy production is oxygen. An abundance of body oxygen results in excellent energy production and a healthy metabolism. A lack of body oxygen results in poor cellular health, an increase in disease conditions and cellular death.

Monocytes: Monocytes are white blood cells that are similar in function to neutrophils (also called phagocytes). The main difference between these two types of white blood cells is that while in the blood stream, they are the immature precursors to phagocytes. Monocytes do not fully mature until they enter the tissues where they can grow to as much as five times their original size. Monocytes are long-lived white blood cells, residing in the tissues from several months to as long as seven years, performing their specific protective functions.

- N -

Naturopathy: Naturopathy is believed to be the oldest form of practicing medicine. The term is derived from the Greek word "natura", meaning nature, and "pathos" meaning suffering. Combined together, the word means "nature is used to heal." Naturopathy is a system, practice or science using natural remedies and agencies to heal instead of synthetic drugs, surgeries or non-natural medical practices.

Neutrophils: Neutrophils are white blood cells that are responsible for isolating and killing bacteria that have invaded the body. Also called "phagocytes" (which means to "engulf",) these cells actually appear to surround and swallow bacteria in the blood stream. Though neutrophils' life spans are short, usually just a few days, they are powerful and strategic hunters supporting the immune system.

Oxidation: The process by which an atom or molecule is changed electrically by the addition or subtraction of electrons altering the electro-chemical makeup and function of the original atom or molecule. At the center of all oxidation processes are oxygen atoms.

Oxygen: The most important element for all life. Named by its discoverer Lavoisier from the Greek word "oxygene" meaning "acid" and "gignesthai" meaning "to be born" since he believed that oxygen was the prime ingredient in all acids. Oxygen is a colorless, tasteless gas that comprises as much as 23% of our atmosphere. Oxygen is a critical ingredient in the oxidation of glucose in the cells to form energy. Oxygen is the most abundant of all the elements and combines chemically with more elements than any other. It is the largest component of organic molecules and is crucial in the respiratory process of animals.

Oxygen Starvation: The physiological condition where the body lacks a sufficient supply of oxygen for normal cellular functions. The result is a drastic pH (acid-alkaline) change, poor metabolic functioning, an increase in body toxins and subsequent fatigue, illness, disease and even death.

Oxygen Therapies: Any modality which introduces oxygen and related therapies as part of a health regimen. These therapies can include deep breathing exercises, hydrogen peroxide and oxidative therapies, ozone therapies, hyperbaric oxygen therapies, ionization therapies and the ingestion of oral stabilized oxygen products. Oxygen therapies are considered an alternative approach to health.

Ozone: An allotropic (different) form of oxygen containing three bonded together oxygen atoms (O-O-O or O3). Ozone comes from the Greek word "ozein" which means "to smell" since ozone has a distinctive and peculiar odor which is similar to the smell of chlorine. Ozone is a very active oxidizing agent and reacts with many other atoms, molecules and compounds. It is also an excellent deodorizer and disinfectant that kills most known pathogenic organisms.

- P -

Pathogens (Pathogenic): An organism that causes disease. Pathogenic organisms include viruses, bacteria, yeasts, molds, fungi and parasites. These organisms use the body as the host to provide them with favorable conditions to multiply. The toxins excreted by these organisms, or their consumption of vital nutrients that they require to grow and reproduce, taxes the body's immune system and reduces the body's oxygen levels and thus the body's ability to fight off these invading pathogens.

pH: A chemistry term that denotes the negative logarithm of the concentration of hydrogen ions in gram atoms in a liter of solution. pH is used to express acidity or alkalinity of a solution or material. pH values range from "0" to "14" with "7" representing neutral pH. Numbers less than seven in value are considered acidic and numbers above seven are considered alkaline. The low pH and high pH values indicate substances that could be caustic and thus toxic to the human body.

Plasma (Blood Plasma): The almost clear liquid component of blood that is 95% water. The remaining 5% is dissolved nutrients, waste products from cellular metabolism, proteins and hormones. The nutrients include sugars, fats amino acids, vitamins and minerals.

Platelets: Platelets are special cells in the blood stream that help stop bleeding and also repair damaged blood vessels by sticking to the vessel walls and adhering to each other to form a dam-like structure.

Potassium: Along with calcium and magnesium, potassium plays a major part in maintaining cardiovascular health. Potassium works hand-in-hand with sodium in what is called the "potassium pump" action that transfers nutrients and oxygen into the cells and removes wastes and carbon dioxide from the cells. Potassium lowers blood pressure and reduces the possibility of strokes. A lack of potassium can result in higher blood pressure, edema (excess water) in the tissues and a more rapid heart rate.

Proteins: Proteins are naturally occurring combinations of amino acids which contain carbon, hydrogen, nitrogen, oxygen and usually sulphur. Proteins are the most important constituents of all living cells and a crucial part of the diet of all higher life forms. There are two main types of proteins: (1) fibrous, which are insoluable and form the structural foundations of our hair, skin, tendons, cartilage and muscles; (2) globular proteins, which are soluble and include enzymes, hormones, hemoglobin and antibodies.

- R -

Radiation Therapy: A cancer therapy where X-rays or other rays that produce ionizing radiation are exposed to cancer cells. As this radiation passes through living and healthy tissue, it slows the tissue's development or destroys the tissue altogether. The effects of exposure to radiation depends on the dosage, the time of exposure (length) and the duration (number of days, weeks, months) of the treatment.

Radiation therapy may produce very unpleasant side effects (called radiation sickness) including fatigue, nausea, loss of appetite and vomiting.

Radiation therapy alters or kills both healthy and unhealthy cells. It is not selective.

R.D.A. (*Recommended Daily Allowance*): R.D.A., also called the U.S.R.D.A., is a listing of vitamins and minerals that the Federal Drug Association has established as the level necessary to maintain average health and to prevent nutritional deficiency. These amounts are as follows:

Vitamin A	5,000 IU
Vitamin C	60 mg
Calcium	1,000 mg
Iron	19 mg
Vitamin D	400 IU
Vitamin E	30 IU
Vitamin K	80 mcg
Thiamin (B1)	1.5 mg
Riboflavin (B2)	1.7 mg
Niacin (B3)	20 mg
Vitamin B6	2 mg
Vitamin B12	6 mcg
Folate (Folic Acid)	400 mcg
Biotin	300 mcg
Pantothenic Acid	10 mg
Phosphorus	1,000 mg
Iodine	150 mcg
Magnesium	400 mg
Zinc	15 mg
Selenium	70 mcg
Copper	2 mg
Manganese	2 mg
Chromium	120 mcg

Molybdenum	75 mcg
Chloride	3,400 mg

Red Blood Cells: Doughnut-shaped cells in the plasma whose main purpose is to transport oxygen to the cells of the body and remove carbon dioxide from the same cells. Red blood cells contain the protein hemoglobin which has the remarkable property of holding oxygen captive while the cell traverses the thousands of miles of arteries and capillaries in the body.

- S -

Sodium: One of the essential minerals needed for a healthy body. Sodium plays a strategic role, along with potassium, in moving nutrients and oxygen into the cells and removing waste products and carbon dioxide out of the cell in an ionic pumping action. Contrary to the belief that high concentrations of sodium cause high blood pressure, there appears to be more medical evidence indicating that a deficiency in potassium may be the primary cause of this condition.

Stabilized Oxygen: Stabilized oxygen is a classification of allotropic forms of oxygen that are combined with other atoms that enables the oxygen to become electrically stable in its attachment to the new molecule. Once in this "stable" state, this new compound can be used as a delivery source for the oxygen as a dietary supplement. These stabilized oxygen molecules may be both in a liquid or dry form. Types of stabilized oxygen include hydrogen peroxide (food grade), chlorine dioxide (chlorite), magnesium peroxide, chlorate and the dissolved diatomic (O2) oxygen found in a small number of products. (See Appendix I.)

Sugars: Sugar is one of the two key elements needed for the production of energy in every cell. (The other is oxygen.) Cells derive the sugar they need for "combustion" in creating A.T.P. energy from breaking down carbohydrates into the simplest form of sugar, glucose.

- T -

Trace Mineral (Essential): Minerals that are essential for maintaining optimum health but are not required in large quantities are called essential trace minerals. There are dozens of trace minerals that are important in small amounts to insure normal functioning of metabolism and the immune system.

- V -

Vein: The blood vessels that return to the heart carrying wastes and carbon dioxide are called veins as opposed to arteries which carry oxygen and nutrients to the cells and organs.

Virus: Some have described a virus as a living crystal that changes its form. A virus, as opposed to a bacteria, lives out its life cycle within the cell by invading the cell and changing the cell's DNA to replicate the virus. For this reason it is more difficult to "kill" viri with traditional drugs and therapies because a virus resides inside the cell emerging only when the cell bursts and the new viri invade new cells to reproduce once again. Oxygen appears to be the only totally effective defense against a virus infection.

Vitamins: Vitamins are essential compounds that the body must have for normal cellular metabolism. With few exceptions, (like Vitamin D, for example,) vitamins cannot be manufactured by the body and must be derived from the foods we eat.

There are 13 major vitamins in two categories: (1) fat soluble and (2) water soluble. The fat soluble vitamins, like A, D, E and K, come directly from foods that contain fats. These vitamins are absorbed into the blood stream in the intestines and then stored in fatty tissue (like the liver) until the body needs them. These vitamins are stored and not excreted or eliminated from the body. Water soluble vitamins, like C, B12, B1, B2, B6, panthothenic acid, biotin and folic acid, are derived from vegetables and fruits and are not stored in the body. They must be regularly supplied on a daily basis. Any excesses of these vitamins are excreted or eliminated from the body.

White Blood Cells: The principle role of the white blood cell is to act as the first line of defense in the immune system against infectious organisms that enter the body. These remarkable soldiers fall into three main categories: (1) granulocytes (which include neutrophils, basophils and eosinophils,) (2) monocytes, and (3) lymphocytes (which include T-type and B-Type cells.)

Yeast: Yeast is a class of minute, uni-cellular fungi that function either aerobically or anaerobically within the body. The most serious pathogenic yeast is Candida albicans (see "Candida") which resides in the digestive tract. Normally kept under control by a beneficial microorganism, Acidophilus, Candida can spread whenever the body is low on oxygen, where the body has too high of a level of stored sugars or when the acid balance of the body has been thrown off because of diet or disease.

Candida infections can cause bloating, diarrhea, constipation, burning, gas and cramping. Candida can invade the entire body not just the intestinal and urinary tract.

About the Author

Stephen R. Krauss has over 30 years of executive management experience in sales, manufacturing, marketing, advertising and promotion, wholesale distribution, all on a national and international scale. He has an undergraduate degree in the liberal arts with minor concentrations in biology/life sciences, math computer science, and a graduate degree in education.

Mr. Krauss has been a C.E.O. and executive board member on numerous private and public corporations including Aquagen International, Inc., a pioneering marketing company in the field of oxygen supplements where he was responsible for product development, marketing, sales and shareholder relations. He left Aquagen in 1996 to start his own nutritional consulting and product development company, BIO2 International, Inc.

BIO2 International specializes in developing oxygen based products and stabilized oxygen technology for numerous industries including agricultural, horticultural, aquacultural, water purification, industrial, aquatic, veterinary, health and nutrition, health and beauty (including cosmetic and beauty products) and dental. BIO2's clients include both small entrepreneurial companies as well as fortune 500 companies.

Mr. Krauss is a nationally recognized corporate consultant in the fields of oxygen nutrition, effective team management and marketing. He has been a featured guest on radio talk shows and at national and international conferences discussing oxygen supplementation. He has also worked as a training consultant with many of the Fortune 500 companies as well as colleges and universities throughout the U.S.

Mr. Krauss has written dozens of articles and books in numerous fields and disciplines including his most recent work *Oxygen: Nature's Most Important Dietary Supplement.*

Mr. Krauss lives in San Luis Obispo, California with his wife and two daughters.